Student

Nutrition, Food, and Fitness

Janis P. Meek, Ed.D., CFCS
Consultant and Writer
Norlina, North Carolina

Nutrition, Food, and Fitness Text
by Dorothy F. West, Ph.D.

Publisher
The Goodheart-Willcox Company, Inc.
Tinley Park, Illinois
www.g-w.com

Introduction

This *Student Activity Guide* is designed for use with the text *Nutrition, Food, and Fitness.* It is divided into chapters that correspond to the chapters in the text. By reading the text first, you will have the information you need to complete the activities in this workbook.

You will find a number of types of activities in this guide. Each chapter ends with a "Backtrack Through the Chapter" activity. This activity will help you recall the facts, interpret implications, and apply and practice chapter material. In addition, you will find activities such as crossword puzzles and fill-in-the-blank sentences. These activities will help build your vocabulary by focusing on terms introduced in the text. True and false and multiple choice questions are often used to help you understand and remember text concepts. Such activities usually have specific "right" answers. You can use these activities as review guides when you study for tests and quizzes. Activities such as evaluations and comparisons will ask for opinions and ideas that cannot be judged as "right" or "wrong." These activities are designed to stimulate your thinking and help you apply text information to your daily life.

Try to complete activities without referring to the text. If necessary, you can look at the book again later to respond to any questions you could not answer. At that time, you can also compare the answers you have to the information in the book. Keep in mind that putting more thought into the activities will help you gain more knowledge from them.

Contents

4

Part Six   Making Informed Choices

Making Wellness a Lifestyle

Lifestyle Choices for Wellness

Activity A

Chapter 1

Name _____

Date _____ Period _____

Complete the left side of the chart below by listing lifestyle choices that would contribute to premature death. Complete the right side of the chart by listing choices that would contribute to optimum health. Try to include choices that relate to each of the aspects of wellness—physical health, mental health, and social health. Then answer the questions at the bottom of the page.

Premature Death ←————————————————————————→ **Optimum Health**

_____   _____

_____   _____

_____   _____

_____   _____

_____   _____

_____   _____

_____   _____

_____   _____

1. When should people adopt healthful lifestyle practices? Explain your answer. _____

_____

_____

_____

2. Why do you think some people make lifestyle choices that can lead to premature death? _____

_____

_____

_____

3. Besides making healthful lifestyle choices, what steps can people take to promote good health? _____

_____

_____

_____

Words in Wellness

Name _____

Date_____ Period _____

Use the clues provided to complete the following puzzle with key words associated with wellness.

1. The average length of life of people living in the same environment is called life _____.
2. A suggested answer to a scientific question, which can be tested and verified.
3. (across) The influence people in a person's age and social group have on his or her behavior is called _____ pressure.
3. (down) The fitness of the body is _____ health.
4. A person's satisfaction with his or her looks, lifestyle, and responses to daily events is called quality of _____.
5. The state of the physical world, including the condition of water, air, and food is _____ quality.
6. A basic component of food that nourishes the body.
7. A principle that tries to explain something that happens in nature.
8. Death that occurs due to lifestyle behaviors that lead to a fatal accident or the formation of an avoidable disease is called _____ death.
9. The identification of a disease.
10. The way a person gets along with other people is _____ health.
11. A state of wellness characterized by peak physical, mental, or social well-being is _____ health.
12. The way a person feels about himself or herself, life, and the world is _____ health.
13. The sum of the processes by which a person takes in and uses food substances.
14. The process researchers use to find answers to their questions is called the _____ method.

Behavior Change Contract

Activity C   Name _____

Chapter 1   Date_____ Period _____

Set a goal for improving your health this week. Use the contract below to record your goal and list specific steps you will take to reach it. Each day you complete a step, give yourself a check mark. At the end of the week, evaluate the results of your efforts by answering the questions at the bottom of the page.

Goal for Health Improvement:							
Steps	Sun.	Mon.	Tues.	Wed.	Thurs.	Fri.	Sat.

Evaluation

1. Are you satisfied with the results of your efforts this week? _____ Explain. _____

   _____

2. What factors helped you complete steps as planned? _____

   _____

3. What factors prevented you from completing steps? _____

   _____

4. Do you need to revise your goal or the steps you will take next week to reach it? _____ If so, how?_____

   _____

Evaluating Health and Nutrition Information

Activity D   **Name** _____

Chapter 1   **Date**_____ **Period** _____

Find a recent article about a health and/or nutrition research study. Attach a copy of the article to this page and answer the following questions.

1. Summarize the content and recommendations of the article.

    _____

    _____

    _____

    _____

2. In what publication did the article appear? _____

3. Who wrote the article? _____

    What are the author's credentials? _____

4. Who conducted the research? _____

    What are the researchers' credentials?_____

5. Who funded the research? _____

    What was the funding organization's motivation for supporting this research? _____

    _____

6. What was the gender and age range of the people involved in the study? _____

7. How many people did the researchers study? _____

8. How long did the study last? _____

9. How was the study set up? (What variables were introduced to different study groups? What type of control

    group was used?) _____

    _____

    _____

10. How did the results of this study compare to the results of other studies? _____

    _____

    _____

11. What other studies are being or will be conducted on this subject?_____

    _____

    _____

12. Does reading this article inspire you to make changes in your lifestyle choices? Explain why or why not.

    _____

    _____

Backtrack
Through Chapter 1

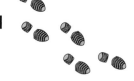

Activity E

Chapter 1

Name _____

Date_____ Period _____

Provide complete answers to the following questions and statements about making wellness a lifestyle choice.

Recall the Facts
- -

1. What are four benefits people might notice when they begin taking steps to improve their health? _____

_____

2. What are the three major components of wellness?_____

_____

3. What is holistic medicine?_____

_____

4. What is a risk factor?_____

_____

5. Name four lifestyle choices that will affect a person's chances of getting a disease._____

_____

6. List three factors that decrease the quality of the environment. _____

_____

7. What is one way patients sometimes interfere with the quality of their health care? _____

_____

8. What are two reasons people develop poor health habits? _____

_____

9. What is epidemiology? _____

_____

10. List three main nutrition problems that are affecting the current state of wellness in the United States._____

_____

Interpret Implications
- -

11. Explain in your own words the difference between mental health and social health._____

_____

12. Why do role expectations sometimes come into conflict? _____

_____

13. Why is the holistic approach considered a good approach to personal health?_____

_____

(Continued)

Name_____

14. Explain the relationship between peer pressure and health habits. _____
_____

15. Why is it often difficult to make changes in personal health habits? _____
_____

16. Explain the relationship between eating habits and life expectancy. _____
_____

Apply & Practice
- -

17. Refer to Figure 1-2 in the text. Where would you place yourself on the wellness continuum today—at the
center, near the "optimum health" end, or near the "premature death" end? _____
What factors caused you to identify this point?_____
_____

18. Give a specific example of how a teen might take a holistic approach to wellness._____
_____
_____

19. If you were concerned about the mental health of a close friend, what would you do?_____
_____
_____

20. Describe a constructive health-related habit you have observed in the life of one of your family members.
_____

Factors Affecting Food Choices

Choices in Context

Activity A

Chapter 2

Name _____

Date_____ Period _____

Read the quotes below about food choices. Identify the factor influencing each choice. Select your answers from the following list:

cultural
religious
social
emotional
historical
media
ethnic
regional
status
individual preference

_____ 1. "Escargot? How can French people bear to eat snails?"

_____ 2. "Mom, let's buy that new Coco-Crunchy cereal we saw on TV."

_____ 3. "The simplest dishes always taste so much better when shared with friends at our potluck suppers!"

_____ 4. "Let's have creamed corn and sweet potatoes like the Pilgrims had for the first Thanksgiving dinner."

_____ 5. "Let's bake some brownies. That will cheer you up."

_____ 6. "We celebrate our holidays with real soul food like turnip greens and ham hocks."

_____ 7. "When I lived in the Southwest, we had tamales every Friday night."

_____ 8. "Mrs. Johnson decided to serve filet mignon because she wanted to impress her new employer."

_____ 9. "I must turn down the prime rib. Like other followers of the Hindu faith, I believe the cow is sacred."

_____ 10. "Buffalo wings are one of my favorites. I like almost anything that is hot and spicy."

How Do Friends Influence Food Choices?

Activity B   **Name** _____

Chapter 2   **Date**_____ **Period** _____

Interview a teen about the influence friends have on his or her food choices. Write the teen's responses to the questions below. Compile your findings with those of your classmates. Then answer the question at the bottom of the page to help you form a conclusion.

Interviewee's age _____   Interviewee's gender _____

1. Other than lunch in the school cafeteria, when was the last time you ate with friends? _____

2. How many people were in your group?_____

3. What brought your group together? _____

4. Where were you? _____

5. Would you have eaten in this location if you had been alone? Explain why or why not. _____

_____

_____

6. What time was it? _____

7. Would you have eaten at this time if you had been alone? Explain why or why not. _____

_____

_____

8. What was your mood?_____

9. What did you talk about while eating? _____

10. Did you eat a meal or a snack? _____

11. What did other people in your group eat?_____

12. What did you eat? _____

13. Would you have eaten the same food if you had been alone? Explain why or why not. _____

_____

_____

14. How might you have improved the nutritional value of your food choices? _____

_____

_____

What role do friends seem to play in influencing what, where, and when teens eat? _____

_____

_____

Food Choice Connection

Activity C

Chapter 2

Name _____

Date_____ Period _____

Match the following terms and definitions.

_____ 1. The application of a certain body of knowledge.

_____ 2. A traditional food of the African American ethnic group.

_____ 3. A belief or attitude that is important to someone.

_____ 4. The beliefs and social customs of a group of people.

_____ 5. A food prepared according to Jewish dietary laws.

_____ 6. A social custom that prohibits the use of certain edible resources as food.

_____ 7. A typical standard or pattern related to food and eating behaviors.

_____ 8. A food that has a social impact on others.

_____ 9. A food that is typical of a given racial, national, or religious culture.

_____ 10. A mainstay food in the diet.

A. culture
B. ethnic food
C. food norm
D. food taboo
E. historical food
F. kosher food
G. soul food
H. staple food
I. status food
J. technology
K. value

Quickly write any mental connections each of the following foods call to your mind. For instance, you might think a given food is fattening, feminine, or healthful. A food might make you think of certain places, events, or groups of people. Compare your mental connections with those of your classmates.

_____ apple

_____ burrito

_____ cheese

_____ cheeseburger

_____ chicken soup

_____ chocolate chip cookie

_____ coffee

_____ fudge

_____ milk

_____ dried plums (prunes)

_____ soda

_____ squash

Food Supply

Activity D   **Name** _____

Chapter 2   **Date** _____ **Period** _____

Choose a specific food item. Use various resources, such as the Internet, library references, and supermarket department managers, to investigate the supply of the item. Look for evidence of how agriculture, technology, economics, and politics have influenced the availability of the selected food. Record your findings and the resources you used in the spaces below.

Food _____

Agriculture

_____

_____

_____

_____

_____

Technology

_____

_____

_____

_____

_____

Economics

_____

_____

_____

_____

_____

Politics

_____

_____

_____

_____

_____

Resources

_____

_____

Backtrack
Through Chapter 2

Activity E

Chapter 2

Name _____

Date_____ Period _____

Provide complete answers to the following questions and statements about factors affecting food choices.

Recall the Facts

1. What are three factors that affect people's food choices? _____
_____

2. What are four factors that help shape culture?_____
_____

3. Who are two groups of people that influenced the cuisine found in the United States today?_____
_____

4. What is an ethnic group? _____
_____

5. What are two reasons people might observe religious food customs?_____
_____

6. What are three ways family members might influence the diets of young eaters?_____
_____

7. What are two types of emotional responses people might have toward food?_____
_____

8. What kinds of problems may be caused by a pattern of using foods for rewards? _____
_____

9. What are four factors that can affect what foods are sold in stores? _____
_____

10. On what is the typical diet of a region usually based? _____
_____

11. What are four decisions political leaders might make that would affect the food supply in a country or region?
_____
_____

12. What sources of nutrition information are most reliable? _____
_____

(Continued)

Name_____

Interpret Implications

13. Why is it important to become aware of how others affect your food choices? _____

_____

14. Why must people examine the way they use food emotionally?_____

_____

15. Explain why a food may taste good to one person but not to another._____

_____

16. How can technological advances in the areas of food production and processing help address the problem

    of world hunger? _____

_____

17. Explain the relationship between economics and the availability of food. _____

_____

_____

Apply & Practice

18. What is an example of a food taboo in your culture? _____

    Would you consider eating this food? Explain why or why not? _____

_____

_____

19. Give an example of a status food._____

    Would you be impressed if someone served you this food? Explain why or why not. _____

_____

_____

20. What is your favorite food commercial? _____

    How has this commercial influenced you? Have you been influenced to buy or try the product? Explain why

    or why not._____

_____

_____

How Nutrients Become You

Food Breakdown

Activity A

Chapter 3

Name _____

Date_____ Period _____

Trace the steps in the process of digestion as food is broken down into simpler substances that can be used by the body. For each step, fill in the blanks with the correct word or words.

Step I: In the Mouth

1. Another word for chewing is

   _____.

2. Good food smells cause secretion of _____.

3. The chemical _____ helps break down food starches.

Step III: In the Stomach

7. The stomach produces _____ juices to help digest food.

8. When these juices combine with food, the result is

   _____.

9. The gastric enzyme that begins to digest protein is

   _____.

Step V: In the Large Intestine

13. Another name for the large intestine is the _____.

14. The main function of the large intestine is to prepare undigested food for _____.

15. Solid wastes that result from digestion are called

    _____.

Step II: In the Esophagus

4. Through the esophagus, food passes from the

   _____ to the

   _____.

5. The _____ prevents swallowed food from entering the windpipe.

6. The squeezing actions of muscles in the esophagus help food move through. This squeezing is known as _____.

Step IV: In the Small Intestine

10. The small intestine has three parts the_____, the

    _____, and the

    _____. Here, about 95 percent of digestion occurs.

11. The pancreas produces

    _____ that break down fats, carbohydrates, and proteins.

12. The liver produces a digestive juice called _____, which aids digestion of fats.

What Could Be Wrong?

Activity B   Name _____

Chapter 3   Date_____ Period _____

In each of the cases below, someone has a gastrointestinal problem. For each case, check each factor that could be affecting digestion and absorption and answer the questions.

Ruth phoned the doctor when her baby, Erica, began vomiting and developed diarrhea. The doctor asked if she had noticed any other symptoms. Then Ruth remembered the skin rash she had seen earlier when she bathed Erica. The doctor asked if Ruth had introduced any new foods into Erica's diet recently. Ruth told the doctor she had fed Erica creamed spinach for the first time that day.

1. Factors: _____ Eating habits _____ Emotions _____ Food allergies _____ Physical activity

2. What could be wrong? _____

_____

3. What should she do? _____

_____

Charla was worried about her calculus grade. She procrastinated about studying for the next test. The night before the test, she studied until 3:00 a.m. She awoke at 7:15 a.m., grabbed a doughnut on the run, and barely made it to class by 8:00. About 45 minutes and four pages of problems later, her stomach twinges had turned into severe pains.

4. Factors: _____ Eating habits _____ Emotions _____ Food allergies _____ Physical activity

5. What could be wrong? _____

_____

6. What should she do? _____

_____

Since he had broken his leg, Derrick hadn't been able to run or play basketball. He was also suffering from chronic indigestion. Derrick couldn't figure out what was causing it. He was eating basically the same amounts of the same foods as before.

7. Factors: _____ Eating habits _____ Emotions _____ Food allergies _____ Physical activity

8. What could be wrong? _____

_____

9. What should he do? _____

_____

Lucas had been eating out a lot lately. Every day for a week, he ate a hamburger, fries, and a milkshake for lunch. He rushed to eat so he could get back to school before sixth period. After each of these meals, Lucas felt stuffed and his stomach was upset.

10. Factors: _____ Eating habits _____ Emotions _____ Food allergies _____ Physical activity

11. What could be wrong? _____

_____

12. What should he do? _____

_____

Digestive Disorders

Activity C

Chapter 3

Name _____

Date _____ Period _____

For each of the following digestive disorders listed below, fill in the needed information. Describe each condition, list one or two causes of the disorder, and identify two treatments or cures available.

Diarrhea

Condition _____

Cause _____

Cure _____

Constipation

Condition _____

Cause _____

Cure _____

Indigestion

Condition _____

Cause _____

Cure _____

Heartburn

Condition _____

Cause _____

Cure _____

(Continued)

Name_____

Ulcer

Condition _____

Cause _____

Cure _____

Gallstones

Condition _____

Cause _____

Cure _____

Diverticulosis

Condition _____

Cause _____

Cure _____

Backtrack
Through Chapter 3

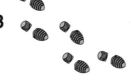

Activity D

Chapter 3

Name _____

Date_____ Period _____

Provide complete answers to the following questions and statements about how the body uses nutrients.

Recall the Facts

1. Of the six types of nutrients, which are elements? _____

   Which are compounds? _____

2. Which three types of nutrients do *not* provide energy? _____

   _____

3. For each of the following functions of nutrients, give an example.

   A. Nutrients build and repair body tissues. _____

   _____

   B. Nutrients regulate all body processes._____

   _____

   C. Nutrients provide energy._____

   _____

4. For each of the following, give the number of calories it provides per gram.

   A. proteins _____

   B. carbohydrates_____

   C. fats _____

   D. alcohol _____

5. Give one example of mechanical digestion and one example of chemical digestion. _____

   _____

6. What is an enzyme? _____

7. What role does the epiglottis play in digestion? _____

8. What is peristalsis? _____

9. How long does food usually remain in the stomach? _____

10. In which part of the body does most digestion take place? _____

11. How long does it take for food to move through the small intestine? _____

12. What does metabolism mean? _____

   _____

(Continued)

Name_____

13. What does ATP stand for and what does it do? _____

_____

14. Identify one way emotions can affect digestion. _____

_____

Interpret Implications

15. Explain the difference between a food allergy and a food sensitivity._____

_____

_____

16. Explain how physical activity affects digestion and absorption. _____

_____

_____

17. Explain why medication is not needed for most digestive disorders. _____

_____

_____

18. Should continuing heartburn be a cause for concern? Why or why not? _____

_____

_____

Apply & Practice

19. Select one personal eating habit you need to improve. Explain how this habit can affect your digestion, absorption, and general wellness._____

_____

_____

_____

_____

_____

20. List three to four tips for managing emotions to avoid digestive problems. _____

_____

_____

_____

_____

_____

Tools for Healthful Eating

Activity A

Chapter 4

Name _____

Date_____ Period _____

Read the following statements about tools for planning a healthful diet. Circle *T* if the statement is true. Circle *F* if the statement is false.

T   F   1. RDAs are suggested levels of nutrients to meet the needs of most healthy people.

T   F   2. RDA stands for *Recommended Daily Allowances.*

T   F   3. RDAs are available for every known nutrient.

T   F   4. The EAR of a nutrient is the recommendation estimated to meet the need of half the healthy people in a group.

T   F   5. The UL is the amount of a nutrient you should consume every day.

T   F   6. The MyPyramid system includes the four basic food groups.

T   F   7. MyPyramid recommends that most teens eat six portions from the grains group each day.

T   F   8. Foods with added fats and sugars are located at the top of MyPyramid because they should be used generously.

T   F   9. Serving sizes on food product labels are required by law to be uniform.

T   F 10. The Dietary Guidelines for Americans focus on nutritious diet, healthy weight, adequate exercise, and food safety.

T   F 11. The Dietary Guidelines recommend that teens spend 30 minutes a day in moderate physical activity.

T   F 12. No single food can supply all the nutrients needed for good health.

T   F 13. Diets that are high in fat, saturated fat, and cholesterol are likely to increase risks of heart disease and stroke.

T   F 14. A high intake of sugar can contribute to obesity and tooth decay.

T   F 15. Restricting salt intake may help reduce the risk of developing high blood pressure.

T   F 16. Children, adolescents, pregnant and breast-feeding women, and alcoholics should refrain from drinking any alcoholic beverages.

T   F 17. Daily Values on food labels are based on a 2,000-calorie diet.

T   F 18. Nutrient density is a comparison of the nutrients in a food with the calories in a food.

T   F 19. A food can have high density for one nutrient and low density for another.

T   F 20. If you do not have a computer, you cannot do diet analysis.

Snack Inspection

Activity B	**Name** _____	
Chapter 4	**Date** _____ **Period** _____	

Compare the nutritional value of four familiar snack foods—potato chips, pretzels, tortilla chips, and a snack mix made from nuts and dried fruit. Before reading the food labels, make predictions about the nutritional value of these snacks. In the middle column of the chart below, record your predictions. Then inspect the food labels to complete the third column. Finally, write your conclusions in the space provided at the bottom of the page.

	Prediction	Inspection
1. Fewest calories		
2. Most calories		
3. Lowest sodium		
4. Lowest total fat		
5. Lowest sugar		
6. Highest saturated fat		
7. Highest trans fat		
8. Highest cholesterol		
9. Highest dietary fiber		
10. Highest protein		
11. Highest vitamin C		
12. Highest calcium		
13. Highest iron		

Conclusions:

_____

_____

_____

_____

(Continued)

Food Labels

Potato Chips

Nutrition Facts
Serving Size 1 oz. (28g/About 17 chips)
Servings Per Container 14

Amount Per Serving

Calories 160   Calories from Fat 90

% Daily Value*

Total Fat 10g	**16%**
Saturated Fat 2g	**15%**
Trans Fat 0g	
Cholesterol 0mg	**0%**
Sodium 180mg	**8%**
Total Carbohydrate 14g	**5%**
Dietary Fiber 1g	**5%**
Sugars 0g	
Protein 2g	

Vitamin A	0%	Vitamin C	10%
Calcium	0%	Iron	0%

* Percent Daily Values are based on a 2,000 calorie diet. Your daily values may be higher or lower depending on your calorie needs:

	Calories	2,000	2,500
Total Fat	Less than	65g	80g
Sat Fat	Less than	20g	25g
Cholesterol	Less than	300mg	300mg
Sodium	Less than	2,400mg	2,400mg
Total Carbohydrate		300g	375g
Fiber		25g	30g

Calories per gram:
Fat 9   Carbohydrates 4   Protein 4

Pretzels

Nutrition Facts
Serving Size 1 oz. (28g/about 48 pretzels)
Servings Per Container 10

Amount Per Serving

Calories 110   Calories from Fat 0

% Daily Value*

Total Fat 0g	**0%**
Saturated Fat 0g	**0%**
Trans Fat 0g	
Cholesterol 0mg	**0%**
Sodium 530mg	**22%**
Total Carbohydrate 23g	**8%**
Dietary Fiber 1g	**3%**
Sugars 1g	
Protein 3g	

Vitamin A	0%	Vitamin C	0%
Calcium	0%	Iron	8%

* Percent Daily Values are based on a 2,000 calorie diet. Your daily values may be higher or lower depending on your calorie needs:

	Calories	2,000	2,500
Total Fat	Less than	65g	80g
Sat Fat	Less than	20g	25g
Cholesterol	Less than	300mg	300mg
Sodium	Less than	2,400mg	2,400mg
Total Carbohydrate		300g	375g
Fiber		25g	30g

Calories per gram:
Fat 9   Carbohydrates 4   Protein 4

Tortilla Chips

Nutrition Facts
Serving Size 1 oz. (28g/About 6 chips)
Servings Per Container 9

Amount Per Serving

Calories 130   Calories from Fat 50

% Daily Value*

Total Fat 6g	**9%**
Saturated Fat 1g	**9%**
Trans Fat 0g	
Cholesterol 0mg	**0%**
Sodium 80mg	**3%**
Total Carbohydrate 19g	**6%**
Dietary Fiber 1g	**5%**
Sugars 0g	
Protein 2g	

Vitamin A	0%	Vitamin C	0%
Calcium	4%	Iron	0%

* Percent Daily Values are based on a 2,000 calorie diet. Your daily values may be higher or lower depending on your calorie needs:

	Calories	2,000	2,500
Total Fat	Less than	65g	80g
Sat Fat	Less than	20g	25g
Cholesterol	Less than	300mg	300mg
Sodium	Less than	2,400mg	2,400mg
Total Carbohydrate		300g	375g
Fiber		25g	30g

Calories per gram:
Fat 9   Carbohydrates 4   Protein 4

Snack Mix

Nutrition Facts
Serving Size ¼ cup (32g)
Servings Per Container 6

Amount Per Serving

Calories 170   Calories from Fat 90

% Daily Value*

Total Fat 11g	**17%**
Saturated Fat 3g	**15%**
Trans Fat 0g	
Polyunsaturated Fat 4g	
Monosaturated Fat 4g	
Cholesterol 0mg	**0%**
Sodium 80mg	**5%**
Potassiuum 115mg	**3%**
Total Carbohydrate 14g	**5%**
Dietary Fiber 2g	**6%**
Sugars 8g	
Protein 4g	

Vitamin A	0%	Vitamin C	2%
Calcium	2%	Iron	4%

Personal Pyramid

Activity C

Chapter 4

Name _____

Date _____ **Period** _____

For each band of the pyramid below, write in the name of the food group or oils category represented. Based on a 2,000-calorie diet, write in the recommended daily amounts for each of the five food groups. Then, list three of your favorite foods from each. Also, record the number of minutes of daily physical activity recommended for teenagers.

Name: _____

Amount: _____

Favorites:

1. _____

2. _____

3. _____

Name: _____

Amount: _____

Favorites:

1. _____

2. _____

3. _____

Name: _____

Amount: _____

Favorites:

1. _____

2. _____

3. _____

Name: _____

Amount: _____

Favorites:

1. _____

2. _____

3. _____

Name: _____

Favorites:

1. _____

2. _____

3. _____

Name: _____

Amount: _____

Favorites:

1. _____

2. _____

3. _____

Daily activity minutes recommended: _____

Backtrack
Through Chapter 4

Activity D

Chapter 4

Name _____

Date _____ Period _____

Provide complete answers to the following questions and statements about nutrition guidelines.

Recall the Facts

1. What does each of the following tell you about a nutrient?

   A. RDA_____

   B. EAR_____

   C. AI_____

   D. UL _____

2. What group issues the DRIs? _____

3. List the names of the food groups in the MyPyramid system. For each group, give the number of portions needed daily for a 2,000 calorie plan. _____

   _____

   _____

   _____

4. What does the width of the food group band in the MyPyramid represent?_____

   _____

5. According to the MyPyramid system, on what does the number of portions needed depend? _____

   _____

6. What do you need to know about portions when following a food plan? _____

   _____

7. List ten of the Dietary Guidelines for Americans. _____

   _____

   _____

   _____

   _____

8. What information does the Daily Value on a nutrition label give?_____

   _____

9. What is nutrient density?_____

   _____

10. Why would a food diary be a useful tool?_____

    _____

(Continued)

Name_____

11. How can you use a computer to analyze your diet? _____
_____

12. How can you use the MyPyramid system in meal planning? _____
_____
_____

Interpret Implications

13. Explain how the DRIs can be used in diet planning. _____
_____

14. Explain how monitoring portion sizes can help you eat more healthfully._____
_____

15. How do variety, balance, and moderation contribute to a healthful diet? _____
_____
_____

16. Explain why descriptions of nutrient density are more useful than the terms *junk food* and *health food* in describing the quality of a food. _____
_____
_____

17. Explain why someone might want to use diet analysis. _____
_____
_____

Apply & Practice

18. For which group or groups from the MyPyramid are you most likely to have trouble eating the recommended number of portions? Why? _____
_____
_____

19. Select a Dietary Guideline for which you need greatest improvement. List four specific actions you could take to better meet this Guideline.
_____
_____
_____

20. Use the MyPyramid system to plan a one-day menu featuring meals and snacks that meet your nutrient needs. Write in the menu below, making sure to include all needed portions from each group.
_____
_____
_____

Carbohydrates: The Preferred Body Fuel

Carbohydrates in Action

Activity A

Chapter 5

Name _____

Date_____ Period _____

Complete the chart below by identifying what type of carbohydrate each item in the first column is. Then list an example where each of the carbohydrates is found.

Carbohydrate	Type (mono-, di-, or polysaccharide)	Where is it found?
1. fiber		
2. fructose		
3. galactose		
4. glucose		
5. lactose		
6. maltose		
7. starch		
8. sucrose		

Plan an advertisement for a food product that is a good source of complex carbohydrates. Be creative as you answer the questions and follow the guidelines below.

What is the name of your product? _____

What is the age and gender of your intended audience? _____

Why do you think your ad will appeal to this audience? _____

_____

In what form of media will your ad appear? (billboards, radio, TV, newspapers, magazines, other)_____

What attention-grabbing phrase or visual image will you use to open your advertisement? _____

_____

Write the main body of your ad. Be sure to explain the important functions of carbohydrates as reasons people should buy your product. _____

_____

_____

What slogan will you use at the end of your ad to help people remember your product? _____

_____

Using Carbohydrates

Activity B   Name _____

Chapter 5   Date_____ Period _____

Write the letter of the answer that best completes each statement in the space provided.

_____ 1. All carbohydrates must be in the form of _____ for cells to use them as an energy source.
   A. fructose   B. glucose

_____ 2. The digestive system _____ poly- and disaccharides from foods.
   A. assembles   B. breaks down

_____ 3. Monosaccharides travel through the _____ to the liver.
   A. bloodstream   B. intestines

_____ 4. The liver converts fructose and galactose into _____.
   A. fat   B. glucose

_____ 5. After a person eats, the amount of glucose in his or her blood _____.
   A. rises   B. falls

_____ 6. Insulin is released by the _____.
   A. liver   B. pancreas

_____ 7. Insulin helps the body _____ blood glucose to a normal level.
   A. raise   B. lower

_____ 8. Insulin triggers body cells to _____ glucose.
   A. burn   B. produce

_____ 9. If cells do not have immediate energy needs, they convert glucose to _____.
   A. glycogen   B. starch

_____10. The muscles store glycogen for use during _____.
   A. muscular activity   B. rest

_____11. The liver stores _____ of the body's glycogen.
   A. one-third   B. two-thirds

_____12. The liver can store a _____ amount of glycogen.
   A. limitless   B. limited

_____13. When someone eats more carbohydrates than the body can immediately use or store as glycogen, the liver will convert the excess into _____.
   A. fat   B. protein

_____14. Fat stores _____ be converted into glucose.
   A. can   B. cannot

Meeting Carbohydrate Needs

Activity C   Name _____

Chapter 5   Date_____ Period _____

Complete the chart below by listing all the foods you ate during one day from each of the indicated groups. Refer to Chart 4-5 in the text for a reminder of how much food equals a portion. Then write the total number of portions from each group in the space below the chart. Complete each equation to determine the approximate number of grams of carbohydrate you consumed from each group. Add the products of all the equations to determine the approximate number of grams of carbohydrate you consumed during the day. Then answer the questions at the bottom of the page.

Breads, Cereals, Rice, and Pasta
Starchy Vegetables (corn, potatoes, winter squash)
Other Vegetables

Fruits
Milk and Yogurt
Legumes
Other Carbohydrates (sugar, jam, jelly, syrup, gelatin)
Regular Soft Drinks

	Total Servings		Grams of Carbohydrate per Serving		
breads	_____	×	15	=	_____
starchy vegetables	_____	×	15	=	_____
other vegetables	_____	×	5	=	_____
fruits	_____	×	15	=	_____
milk and yogurt	_____	×	12	=	_____
legumes	_____	×	15	=	_____
other carbohydrates	_____	×	15	=	_____
soft drinks	_____	×	36	=	_____

Total grams of carbohydrate consumed   _____

How did your carbohydrate consumption compare to the daily recommendation of 250 to 300 grams, which is appropriate for most teens? _____

Most people in the United States need to decrease their intake of refined sugars and increase their intake of complex carbohydrates. How could you accomplish these goals? _____

_____

Fuel for the Body

Name _____

Date_____ Period _____

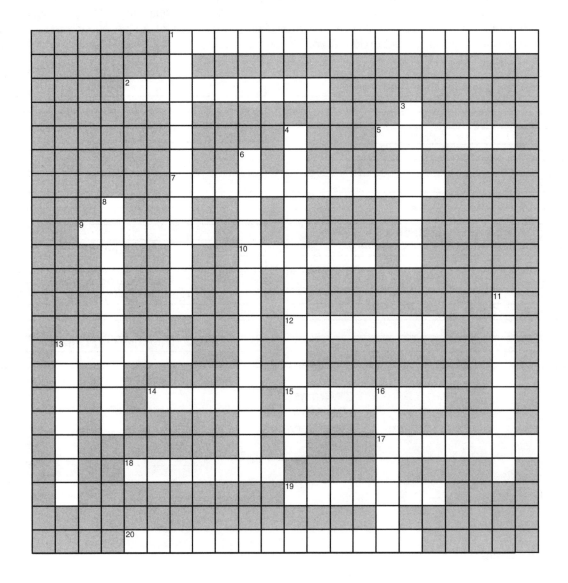

Name_____

Across

1. A lack of or an inability to use the hormone insulin.
2. An indigestible carbohydrate from plants that does not dissolve in water is _____ fiber.
5. Tooth decay is called dental _____.
7. A low blood glucose level.
9. A collective term used to refer to all the monosaccharides and disaccharides.
10. A polysaccharide that is the storage form of energy in plants.
12. A chemical produced in the body and released into the bloodstream to regulate specific body processes.
13. Monosaccharides and disaccharides are known as _____ carbohydrates.
14. Indigestible polysaccharides that make up the tough, fibrous cell walls of plants.
15. A hormone secreted by the pancreas to regulate blood glucose level.
17. Polysaccharides, such as starch and fiber, are called _____ carbohydrates.
18. A carbohydrate sweetener that is separated from its natural source for use as a food additive is called _____ sugar.
19. A monosaccharide that circulates in the bloodstream and serves as the body's source of energy.
20. One of the six classes of nutrients that includes sugars, starches, and fibers.

Down

1. A carbohydrate made up of two sugar units.
3. The feeling of fullness a person has after eating food.
4. A carbohydrate made up of many sugar units that are linked in straight or branched chains.
6. A carbohydrate made up of single sugar units.
8. A concentrated source of a nutrient, usually in pill, liquid, or powder form.
11. The body's storage form of glucose.
13. An indigestible carbohydrate from plants that dissolves in water is _____ fiber.
16. An inability to digest the main carbohydrate in milk due to a lack of the digestive enzyme lactase is called _____ intolerance.

Carbohydrate Headlines

Name _____

Date_____ Period _____

These tabloid headlines represent some common myths about the effects of carbohydrates in the diet. Use the space provided to write a brief rebuttal debunking each myth.

Starchy Foods Add Pounds and Inches Unlimited

_____
_____
_____

Lay Off Sweets or Lose Your Teeth!

_____
_____
_____

Kids + Sugar = HYPER!

_____
_____
_____

Sugar? Give In and Get Addicted…

_____
_____
_____

In Go the Sweets, Up Goes the Glucose—Look Out, Diabetes!

_____
_____
_____

Backtrack
Through Chapter 5

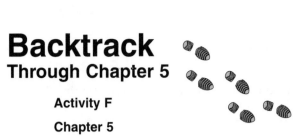

Activity F

Chapter 5

Name _____

Date_____ Period _____

Provide complete answers to the following questions and statements about carbohydrates.

Recall the Facts

1. What three components of the diet are supplied by carbohydrates? _____
   _____

2. Of what three chemical elements are carbohydrates composed? _____

3. What happens to disaccharides during digestion? _____
   _____

4. What are four foods that are high in simple carbohydrates and four foods that are high in complex carbohydrates?

   simple: _____

   complex: _____

5. What are the four key functions served by carbohydrates? _____
   _____
   _____

6. What are three diseases that may be prevented or controlled by fiber in the diet? _____
   _____

7. What are the two categories of sugars in foods? _____
   _____

8. What percent of daily calories should come from refined sugars?_____
   What percent should come from complex carbohydrates?_____

9. How many calories are provided by a gram of carbohydrates? _____

10. What are six symptoms of diabetes mellitus?_____
    _____
    _____

Interpret Implications

11. Why are carbohydrates known as the body's preferred source of energy? _____
    _____

12. How does carbohydrate consumption relate to the body's use of proteins? _____
    _____
    _____

(Continued)

Name_____

13. How does fiber help prevent constipation, reduce the likelihood of hemorrhoids, and relieve diarrhea?_____
    _____
    _____

14. If the body converts all carbohydrates to glucose anyway, why do experts recommend eating more complex carbohydrates than simple sugars? _____
    _____
    _____

15. How can you identify foods that are high in refined sugars? _____
    _____

16. Why would a dentist advise a patient to avoid snacking on sugars and starches between meals?_____
    _____
    _____

17. How might someone who is lactose intolerant meet his or her need for calcium?_____
    _____

Apply & Practice

18. How many grams of fiber should you include in your diet each day?_____

19. Imagine you are giving a birthday party for a young child. Several parents express concern about their children coming home hyperactive from all the sweets eaten at the party. How will you address these concerns? _____
    _____
    _____

20. A friend tells you he thinks he has hypoglycemia because he gets a headache and feels shaky every afternoon. How would you respond? _____
    _____
    _____

Fats: A Concentrated Energy Source

Facing Fats

Activity A

Chapter 6

Name _____

Date _____ Period _____

Fill in the chart below describing types of fat, the prevalent types of fatty acids they contain, and their states at room temperature. Then answer the questions at the bottom of the page about triglycerides and other lipids.

Type of Fat	Prevalent Type of Fatty Acid	State at Room Temperature
1. beef fat		
2. corn oil		
3. olive oil		
4. soybean oil		
5. lard		
6. tropical oils		
7. peanut oil		
8. butter		
9. safflower oil		

10. Why would a manufacturer want to use hydrogenation? _____

_____

_____

11. Are trans-fatty acids better for you than saturated fatty acids? Why or why not? _____

_____

_____

12. What is a phospholipid? _____

13. Where is lecithin found? _____

14. Why are emulsifiers used? _____

15. Name two uses for cholesterol in the body. _____

_____

16. Which has more cholesterol—vegetable oil or animal fat? Why? _____

_____

What's My Job?

Activity B   Name _____

Chapter 6   Date_____ Period _____

Fill in the chart by listing six functions that lipids perform in the body. In the second column, give an example of each function.

Function	Example
1.	1.
2.	2.
3.	3.
4.	4.
5.	5.
6.	6.

Each "clue" below describes a part of a process involving lipids in the body. Match each clue with the appropriate term.

_____ 1. If fat is needed by the body, I break it down for immediate use. If fat is not needed right away, I convert it back to triglycerides for storage.

_____ 2. I act as an emulsifier, breaking fat into tiny droplets that can be suspended in the digestive juices.

_____ 3. I am supplied by the pancreas to break triglycerides into glycerol, fatty acids, and monoglycerides.

_____ 4. I serve as a transport line through which lipids pass on their way to the body cells.

_____ 5. With my protein and phospholipid coat, I can carry fat but be absorbed by the lymphatic system.

_____ 6. Fat mixes with bile inside me.

_____ 7. I pick up cholesterol from around the body and transfer it to other lipoproteins, who return it to the liver.

_____ 8. I carry triglycerides and cholesterol made by the liver to the body cells so they can use them.

_____ 9. I store a limitless supply of triglycerides and send fatty acids through the bloodstream to other body cells for fuel.

_____ 10. I absorb chylomicrons before they enter the bloodstream.

_____ 11. I produce bile and cholesterol. I also process returned cholesterol as a waste product for removal from the body.

_____ 12. I carry cholesterol (not triglycerides) through the bloodstream to the body.

_____ 13. I am one of four special combinations of fat and protein that help transport fats in the body.

A. bile

B. bloodstream

C. body cell

D. chylomicrons

E. enzymes

F. fat cells

G. HDL

H. large intestine

I. LDL

J. lipoproteins

K. liver

L. lymphatic system

M. small intestine

N. VLDL

Recognize the Risks

Activity C   **Name** _____

Chapter 6   **Date**_____ **Period** _____

In each of the following pairs, place an **R** in the blank beside the description of the person with the greater risk for coronary heart disease. Then answer the questions at the bottom of the page.

1. _____twenty-five years old   _____sixty years old
2. _____male   _____female
3. _____African American   _____Asian American
4. _____second cousin had a heart attack   _____father has high blood pressure
5. _____overweight   _____underweight
6. _____chain smoker   _____nonsmoker
7. _____lowfat diet   _____high fat diet
8. _____active lifestyle   _____sedentary lifestyle
9. _____irritable, impatient personality   _____mild personality traits
10. _____low-stress work   _____normal-stress work
11. _____normal blood pressure   _____high blood pressure
12. _____diabetic   _____nondiabetic
13. _____high serum cholesterol   _____low serum cholesterol

14. Of the risk factors listed in the chapter, which are uncontrollable?_____
_____
_____
_____

15. Which are controllable?_____
_____
_____
_____

16. For each risk factor that is controllable, explain what a person could do to lower his or her risk. _____
_____
_____
_____
_____
_____
_____

Heart of the Matter

Activity D

Chapter 6

Name _____

Date _____ Period _____

For each row in the puzzle, write in the correct term from the chapter. Use the numbered clues to help you.

1. A substance, such as a phospholipid, that can mix with water and fat.
2. The death of heart tissue caused by blockage of an artery carrying nutrients and oxygen to that tissue.
3. A fatty acid that forms when oils are partially hydrogenated.
4. A(n) _____ fatty acid has only one double bond between carbon atoms in a carbon atom chain.
5. The body stores lipids in _____ tissue.
6. A fat that has spoiled, giving it an unpleasant smell and taste.
7. Lipids with a phosphorus-containing compound in their chemical structure. They can combine with both fat and water to form emulsions.
8. _____ disease is the name for disease of the heart and blood vessels.
9. A phospholipid made by the liver and found in many foods.
10. _____-3 fatty acids are a type of polyunsaturated fatty acids found in fish oils. They have been shown to have a positive effect on heart health.
11. The body cannot make this type of fatty acid, but it is needed for normal growth and development, so it must be supplied by the diet.
12. A(n) _____ fatty acid has at least one double bond between two carbon atoms in a carbon atom chain and, therefore, is missing at least two hydrogen atoms.
13. Fat droplets that are coated by proteins so they can be transported in the bloodstream.
14. A(n) _____ fatty acid has no double bonds in its chemical structure and, therefore, carries a full load of hydrogen atoms.
15. An organic compound that is made up of a chain of carbon atoms to which hydrogen atoms are attached and has an acid group at one end.
16. A white, waxy lipid made by the body that is part of every cell. It is also found in foods of animal origin.
17. A group of compounds that includes triglycerides, phospholipids, and sterols.
18. A(n) _____ lipoprotein picks up cholesterol from around the body and transfers it to other lipoproteins for transport back to the liver for removal from the body.
19. A(n) _____ fatty acid that has two or more double bonds between carbon atoms in a carbon atom chain.
20. The process of breaking the double carbon bonds in unsaturated fatty acids and adding hydrogen to make the fatty acid more saturated.
21. A(n) _____-density lipoprotein carries triglycerides and cholesterol made by the liver through the bloodstream to the body.
22. The major type of fat found in foods and in the body. It consists of three fatty acids attached to glycerol.
23. Abnormally high blood pressure; an excess force on the walls of the arteries as blood is pumped from the heart.
24. A condition of hardened and narrowed arteries caused by plaque deposits.
25. A medical test that measures the amounts of cholesterol, triglycerides, HDL, and LDL in the blood is a(n) _____ profile.
26. A buildup of fatty compounds made up largely of cholesterol that form on the inside walls of arteries.
27. The death of brain tissue caused by blockage of an artery carrying nutrients and oxygen to that tissue.
28. A ball of triglycerides thinly coated with cholesterol, phospholipids, and proteins formed to carry absorbed dietary fat to body cells.
29. An ingredient used in food products to replace some or all the fat typically found in those products.

(Continued)

Name____________________________________

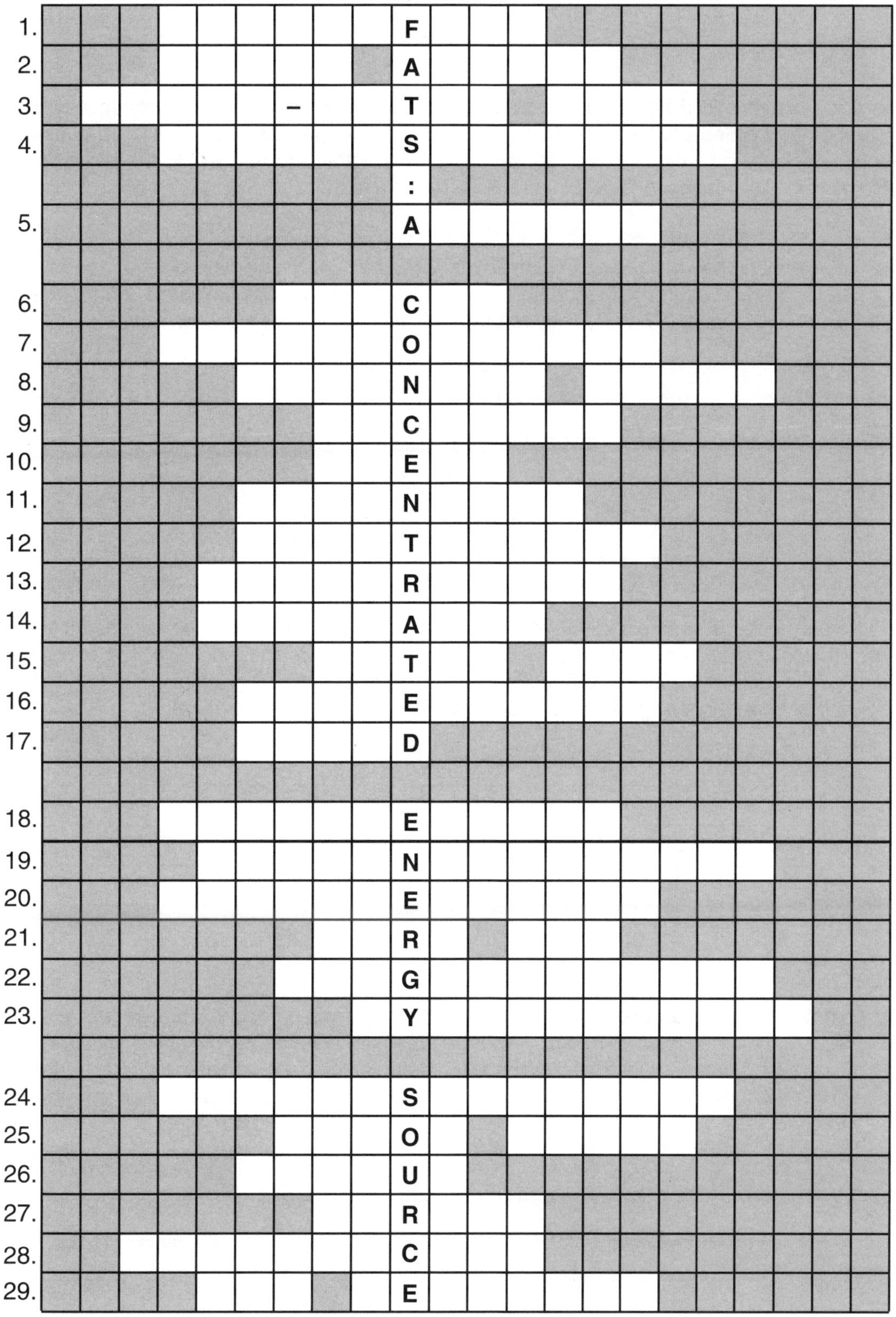
1. F
2. A
3. – T
4. S
:
5. A
6. C
7. O
8. N
9. C
10. E
11. N
12. T
13. R
14. A
15. T
16. E
17. D
18. E
19. N
20. E
21. R
22. G
23. Y
24. S
25. O
26. U
27. R
28. C
29. E

Letters from Lowfat Lane

Activity E	**Name** _____
Chapter 6	**Date** _____ **Period** _____

Pretend you are a community dietitian. You teach nutrition classes for groups in your community. Your last class was at a neighborhood called Lowfat Lane. After your presentation, several people still had questions about fat intake. They have written to you asking your advice. Read each letter and respond to the person's concerns. Be sure your advice is well grounded in factual information from the text.

Dear Dietitian:
I enjoyed your presentation. You persuaded me to make the switch from whole milk to fat free milk in my household. Unfortunately, I haven't been very successful. My husband and sons are giving me a hard time over it. They just don't like the taste of the fat free milk! They refuse to drink it. How can I convince them?
Minus the Milkfat Mom

_____

_____

_____

_____

_____

Dear Dietitian:
My friend, Flora Foster is paranoid about fat. She seems to be going overboard in her search for a fat-free life, though. When she took her son Freddy for his six-week checkup, she asked the pediatrician if he could recommend a fat-free formula. She is worried little Freddy will grow up to be obese like his grandfather. She wants to start right away to prevent that from happening. What do you think about fat-free infant formula?
Flustered over Flora

_____

_____

_____

_____

_____

Dear Dietitian:
My wife Franny and I are planning to host a cookout for the neighborhood this weekend. Our new neighbors are very conscious of their fat intake, so we have planned the menu accordingly. We aren't having steaks, because they have marbling and fat around the edges. Instead, we're serving hot dogs. They offer smaller portions and less visible fat. Since our meal will be so healthful, we plan to serve them with chili, slaw, and all the trimmings! Thanks for your presentation. We're on our way now!
Heart-Healthy Hosts

_____

_____

_____

_____

_____

(Continued)

Name_____

Dear Dietitian:

My cousin Faith is working hard to lose fifty pounds as her doctor recommended. She has cut down her fat intake and kept a daily food diary for the last three months. She seems to be making some progress. When I saw Faith the other day, she said she has lost eight pounds. Her only complaint was that it seemed to be taking forever. I didn't know what to say to her. What do you think? Is there anything I can do to help her?

Concerned Clara

_____
_____
_____
_____
_____

Dear Dietitian:

My husband Fritz took me out to dinner last night. We had grilled chicken, fat-free dressing on the salad, and baked potatoes. We topped it off with the dessert specialty of the house, "Death by Chocolate." We figured it was okay to splurge, since we had eaten such a smart meal! Were we right?

Wondering Wanda

_____
_____
_____
_____
_____

Dear Dietitian:

At your presentation, you briefly mentioned fat replacers. I want to know more about them. Are they safe? Do products that use them taste the same as regular products? Are they lower in calories? Where can I find them?

Inquisitive Irene

_____
_____
_____
_____
_____

Dear Dietitian:

I am trying to eat more healthfully. I have been eating fish instead of higher-fat meats. I found that if I fry the fish in oil and serve it with French fries, it tastes pretty good. When I'm really on top of it, I add a small vegetable salad with lots of salad dressing and cornbread with lots of butter. I'm so glad you advised me to eat more fish. Thanks!

Crazy for Catfish

_____
_____
_____
_____
_____

Backtrack
Through Chapter 6

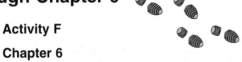

Activity F

Chapter 6

Name _____

Date_____ Period _____

Provide complete answers to the following questions and statements about fats.

Recall the Facts

1. What is the composition of triglycerides? _____
   _____

2. Which fats tend to be higher in saturated fatty acids—those from animals or those from plants?_____

3. What are the two main reasons for hydrogenating oils?_____
   _____

4. Why is lecithin important in the making of homemade mayonnaise?_____
   _____

5. Why are lecithin and cholesterol not essential in the diet?_____
   _____

6. Give three examples of sterols _____

7. How do lipids reach body tissues? _____
   _____

8. What is the leading cause of death in the United States? _____

9. Why do young females tend to have less risk for heart disease than young males?_____
   _____

10. List seven controllable factors that affect heart health._____
    _____
    _____
    _____

11. Name four ways exercise can have a positive effect on heart health. _____
    _____
    _____

12. What is the relationship between fat in the diet and risk for cancer? _____
    _____

(Continued)

Name_____

Interpret Implications

13. Why is the word *lipid* considered broader than the word *fat*? _____

_____

_____

14. Explain the difference between LDL and HDL. _____

_____

_____

15. Explain how plaque buildup in the arteries causes high blood pressure. _____

_____

_____

16. Explain why some cholesterol is termed "good" and some is termed "bad." _____

_____

_____

17. An article reported that native Alaskans who consumed a lot of fish oil had a low rate of CHD. Would it then be wise to conclude taking fish oil pills would reduce the risk of heart attack? Why or why not? _____

_____

_____

_____

Apply & Practice

18. What was the most startling fact you learned about fats from reading the chapter? How will you use this information to help you eat more healthfully? _____

_____

_____

_____

19. Your friend has an overweight mother and a father with high blood pressure. She has gone on a totally fat-free diet because she wants to stay slim and healthy. What advice would you offer her? _____

_____

_____

_____

20. List four ways you can modify your diet to limit fats and cholesterol. _____

_____

_____

_____

Proteins: The Body's Building Blocks

7

Building Blocks of Protein

Activity A

Chapter 7

Name _____

Date _____ Period _____

Choose the best response to complete each multiple choice statement. Write the letter for each answer in the block below containing the same number as the statement. Your answers will reveal an essential component of proteins.

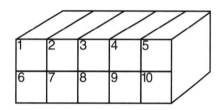

1. Protein differs from carbohydrates and fats because of the _____ it contains.
   A. nitrogen   B. oxygen   C. hydrogen   D. carbon

2. Protein makes up about _____ percent of your body.
   L. 12 to 15   M. 18 to 20   N. 20 to 25   O. 30 to 40

3. When proteins change shape and take on new characteristics, _____ has occurred.
   G. balance   H. completion   I. denaturation   J. coagulation

4. To say the body can synthesize a compound means that it can _____ it.
   L. destroy   M. digest   N. make   O. complement

5. There are _____ essential amino acids.
   L. 20   M. 19   N. 11   O. 9

6. Proteins that defend the body against infection and disease are _____.
   A. antibodies   B. buffers   C. enzymes   D. hormones

7. The liver converts nitrogen waste from proteins into _____.
   A. enzymes   B. lipoproteins   C. urea   D. urine

8. Plants that can capture nitrogen from the air and transfer it to their protein-rich seeds are _____.
   G. grains   H. hummus   I. legumes   J. tofu

9. Complete proteins come from _____ sources.
   A. plant & animal   B. only plant   C. only mineral   D. only animal

10. Two proteins that together provide all essential amino acids are said to be _____.
    Q. complete   R. animal   S. complementary   T. valuable

Copyright Goodheart-Willcox Co., Inc.

49

A Billboard for Proteins

Activity B   Name _____

Chapter 7   Date _____ Period _____

In the space provided below, list the six basic functions of protein in the body. Then design a billboard to advertise one of the functions. Choose a function and write a summary of the message of your design. Use the box at the bottom of the page to illustrate your billboard. Be sure to use an attention-getting slogan, logo, and layout.

Functions of Protein

1. _____   4. _____

2. _____   5. _____

3. _____   6. _____

Summary of Message

_____

_____

_____

Animal vs. Plant Proteins

Activity C

Chapter 7

Name _____

Date_____ Period _____

Complete the following chart to contrast plant and animal proteins. Supply the information called for in each row of the chart. Then answer the question at the bottom of the page.

	Animal Sources	Plant Sources
Examples		
Quality		
Advantages		
Disadvantages		

Do you choose more protein from plant sources or animal sources? Explain your response.

_____

_____

_____

Complementary Proteins—A "Good Match"

Activity D

Chapter 7

Name _____

Date _____ Period _____

Circle the ingredients in the two recipes below that are complementary sources of protein. Use a recipe book to find a third example of a recipe containing complementary proteins. Write the name of the recipe on the tab of the third recipe card below. List the ingredients for the recipe on the lines of the card. Then circle the complementary sources of protein contained in the recipe.

Vegetarian Chili Mac

3   cups canned tomatoes
¾ cup uncooked macaroni
¾ cup chopped onion
2   cloves garlic, crushed
¼ cup chopped green pepper

1   tablespoon oil
2   teaspoons chili powder
1   teaspoon dried basil
3   cups canned kidney beans

Stir-Fried Vegetables and Tofu

1   cup orange-ginger sauce
2   tablespoons peanut oil
1   medium onion
2   carrots
2   ribs celery

2   cups broccoli florets
1   medium red bell pepper
½ pound mushrooms
1   cup bean sprouts
1½ cups diced firm tofu
6   cups cooked brown rice

_____

_____

_____

_____

_____

_____

_____

_____

Protein Balance

Activity E

Chapter 7

Name _____

Date_____ Period _____

Decide which of the following statements about protein needs are true and which are false. Write the numbers of statements that are true inside the blocks on the left end of the scale. Write the numbers of those that are false on the right end. If you have identified the statements correctly, you will have the same number on each end, thus preserving the "protein balance."

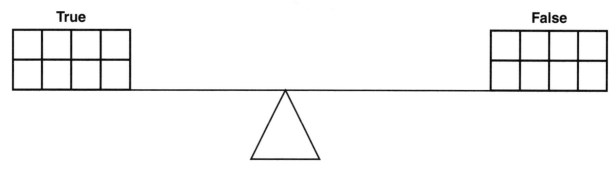

1. The human body stores excess protein for future needs.

2. The amount of protein a person needs is related to his or her activity level.

3. Most people in the United States eat more protein than they need.

4. Children need proportionally more protein than adults.

5. Extra protein is needed to support the growth of unborn babies in pregnant women and the production of milk in breast-feeding mothers.

6. In general, females require more protein than men of the same age and size.

7. A large, tall person needs more protein than a small, short person.

8. Sick people require extra protein to build antibodies.

9. The RDAs for protein include a margin of safety.

10. To meet the RDA, approximately 20 percent of daily calories should come from protein.

11. The Nutrition Facts panel on food products can help people estimate how much protein they consume each day.

12. People who exercise occasionally need extra protein to build muscle and supply energy.

13. Athletes should consume more calories from protein than from carbohydrates.

14. The grains and vegetable groups of the MyPyramid system are the primary food sources of protein.

15. One-fourth cup of cooked legumes equals one ounce of meat.

16. People can avoid health risks by choosing protein sources that are high in saturated fats.

Not Too Little—Not Too Much

Activity F　　　　　　　　Name _____

Chapter 7　　　　　　　　Date_____ Period _____

Use the clues provided to identify conditions brought on by too little or too much protein in the diet. Write one letter in each space. Note the first four answers are in the "plus zone," reflecting too much protein intake. The last four answers are in the "minus zone," reflecting too little protein intake.

"Plus Zone"

1. _ _ _ _ _ _ _
2. _ _ _ _ _ _ _ _ _ _ _
3. _ _ _ _ _ _ _ _ _ _ _ _ _ _
4. _ _ _ _ _ _ _ _ _ _ _ _ _ _ _ _ _ _ _ _ _

Protein • Protein • Protein • Protein • Protein • Protein • Protein • Protein • Protein• Protein

5. _ _ _ _ _ _ - _ _ _ _ _ _ _ _ _ _ _ _ _ _ _ _ _ _
6. _ _ _ _ _ _ _ _ _ _ _ _ _ _ _ _ _ _ _ _ _ _ _
7. _ _ _ _ _ _ _ _ _ _
8. _ _ _ _ _ _ _ _

"Minus Zone"

1. Since many high-protein foods are also high-fat foods, the result of a high-protein diet may be excess _____ _____.

2. When a person consumes a high-protein diet from animal sources, he or she may develop _____ _____ in the bones.

3. A high-protein diet creates extra work for the _____ _____ _____, the organs responsible for handling nitrogen waste.

4. A person who takes in more protein than he or she excretes is in _____ _____ _____.

5. A lack of calories and proteins in the diet causes a condition called _____ -_____ _____.

6. A person who loses more nitrogen than he or she consumes is in _____ _____ _____.

7. When mothers in poor countries wean older children to begin breast-feeding newborns, the older children may develop _____.

8. The muscles and tissues of people suffering from starvation begin to waste away due to a PEM disease called _____.

Backtrack
Through Chapter 7

Activity G

Chapter 7

Name _____

Date_____ Period _____

Provide complete answers to the following questions and statements about proteins.

Recall the Facts

- -

1. Of what four elements are proteins composed? _____

   _____

2. What are four factors or substances that can denature proteins? _____

   _____

3. How many amino acids are needed for good health? _____ How many of the amino acids are essential? _____ How many are nonessential? _____

4. What are six functions of proteins in the body? _____

   _____

   _____

5. What are three important compounds the body makes from proteins? _____

   _____

6. What are three vital substances that are carried by proteins in the bloodstream?_____

   _____

7. What are four factors that influence protein food choices?_____

   _____

   _____

8. Name six types of legumes. _____

   _____

9. What are three positive factors associated with plant sources of protein in terms of heart health and cancer risk reduction?_____

   _____

   _____

10. What four factors determine the amount of protein you need?_____

    _____

    _____

11. What groups of the MyPyramid system are the primary food sources of protein?_____

    _____

12. What population group is often affected by kwashiorkor? _____

    _____

(Continued)

Name_____

Interpret Implications

13. Explain why adults need dietary protein even though they have reached their growth potential. _____

_____

14. Explain why proteins are not considered the preferred source of body energy._____

_____

_____

15. Explain the difference between complete proteins and incomplete proteins. _____

_____

_____

16. How can an athlete meet added needs for protein? _____

_____

17. Why is nitrogen balance used to evaluate a person's protein status? _____

_____

Apply & Practice

18. What protein source would you choose to complement whole grain bread when serving lunch to a vegetarian friend? Explain your choice. _____

_____

_____

19. What is your RDA for protein?_____

20. Suppose your friend is a body builder. He tells you he has been following a high-protein diet and consuming amino acid supplements to help increase his muscle mass. Describe and explain your response._____

_____

_____

_____

Vitamins: Drivers of Cell Processes

8

Vitamin Analogies

Activity A   Name _____

Chapter 8   Date_____ Period _____

For each analogy given, underline the term from the parentheses that best completes the analogy. (An *analogy* is a comparison between two sets of concepts. For example, "vitamins : body processes :: thermostat : room temperature" is read "vitamins are to body processes as a thermostat is to room temperature." This analogy means vitamins regulate body processes just as thermostats regulate room temperatures.)

1. provitamin : vitamin :: beta-carotene : (thiamin, vitamin A, vitamin C, vitamin D)

2. fat-soluble : vitamins A, D, E and K :: water-soluble : (thiamin and riboflavin, folate and niacin, B-complex and vitamin C, biotin and thiamin)

3. food poisoning : foodborne bacteria :: toxicity : (large doses of supplements, vitamin deficiencies, undernourishment, malabsorption)

4. epithelial : human body :: (windows, siding, flooring, plumbing) : house

5. riboflavin : inflamed tongue :: vitamin A : (crossed eyes, night blindness, cataracts, glaucoma)

6. Basic Four : MyPyramid :: micrograms : (beta-carotene, carotene equivalent, provitamin, retinol equivalent)

7. enriched : breads :: fortified : (cereals, vegetables, dairy products, meats)

8. children : adults :: rickets : (osteomalacia, osteoporosis, skin cancer, heart disease)

9. (vitamin A, vitamin C, vitamin D, vitamin K) : osteomalacia :: calcium : osteoporosis

10. antioxidant : protection from oxygen exposure :: free radical : (tissue growth, tissue damage, tissue exposure, tissue transformation)

11. folate deficiency : neural tube :: erythrocyte hemolysis : (plasma, white blood cells, red blood cells, iron)

12. incineration : burning :: coagulation : (bleeding, hemorrhaging, clotting, bandaging)

13. players : team :: B vitamins : (provitamins, coenzymes, enzymes, complex)

14. alcoholism : thiamin :: smoking : (vitamin A, vitamin C, vitamin D, vitamin K)

15. scurvy : vitamin C :: beriberi : (thiamin, riboflavin, niacin, biotin)

16. niacin flush : toxicity :: (pellagra, pernicious anemia, rickets, erythrocyte hemolysis) : deficiency

17. cement : bricks :: (plasma, antioxidant, collagen, choline) : cells

18. pellagra : flaky skin :: pernicious anemia : (vitality, dry mouth, skin tingling, dementia)

Vitamin Sources and Functions

Activity B   Name _____

Chapter 8   Date_____ Period _____

Use a food composition table or other reliable source to complete the chart below. For each vitamin, list foods that are good sources of the vitamin. Then list functions of the vitamin in the body, the classification (whether the vitamin is fat-soluble or water-soluble), and the RDA or AI recommendation for someone of your age and gender.

Vitamin	Food Sources	Functions	Classification	RDA or AI
1. biotin				
2. folate				
3. niacin				
4. pantothenic acid				
5. riboflavin				
6. thiamin				
7. vitamin A				
8. vitamin B_6				
9. vitamin B_{12}				
10. vitamin C				
11. vitamin D				
12. vitamin E				
13. vitamin K				

Cause and Effect

Activity C

Chapter 8

Name _____

Date_____ Period _____

Fill in the missing information to complete the chart below. In some cases, you will need to provide the cause of the problem that is given. In other cases, you will list the effect of the deficiency or excess given.

Cause	Effect
1.	1. Night blindness
2.	2. Beriberi
3. Riboflavin deficiency	3.
4.	4. Rickets
5. Vitamin E deficiency in babies	5.
6.	6. Abnormal heart rhythms
7. Excess vitamin A	7.
8. Large doses of vitamin B_6	8.
9.	9. Jaundice
10. Folate deficiency	10.
11.	11. Pellagra
12. Inability to absorb vitamin B_{12}	12.
13. Vitamin D excess	13.
14.	14. Scurvy
15. Toxic levels of niacin	15.
16. Megadoses of vitamin C	16.

Foods vs. Supplements

Activity D   Name _____

Chapter 8   Date_____ Period _____

Use the space provided to compare and contrast the benefits of getting vitamins from supplements with those of getting vitamins from food sources.

Benefits of Vitamin Supplements

_____

_____

_____

_____

_____

_____

_____

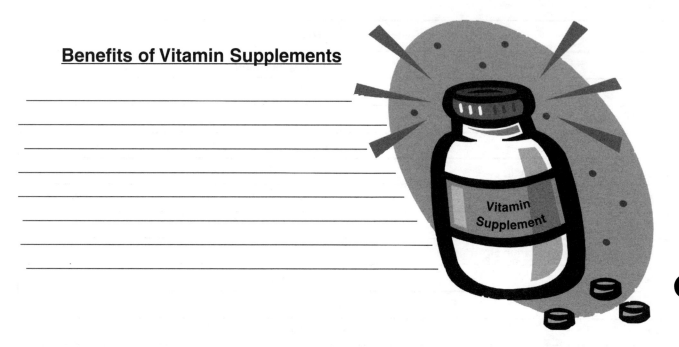

Benefits of Vitamins from Foods

_____

_____

_____

_____

_____

_____

Viva Las Vitamins!

Activity E   Name _____

Chapter 8   Date_____ Period _____

"Long live the vitamins!" Except in special circumstances, a balanced diet supplies all the vitamins needed by the body. Unfortunately, many vitamins are needlessly lost due to poorly chosen methods for food selection, preparation, and storage. Use the boxes provided to design mini-posters about preservation of vitamins in foods.

Food Selection

(Continued)

Name_____

Food Preparation

Food Storage

Backtrack
Through Chapter 8

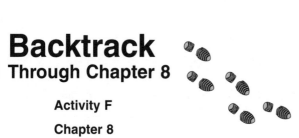

Activity F

Chapter 8

Name _____

Date _____ Period _____

Provide complete answers to the following questions and statements about vitamins.

Recall the Facts

1. How many calories per gram do vitamins provide? _____

2. Why does the body need vitamins? _____

3. What makes vitamins organic compounds? _____

    _____

4. How long does it usually take for a vitamin deficiency to produce first symptoms? _____

5. Name three stages in the life cycle during which the body has a greater than usual need for vitamins. _____

    _____

6. What is toxicity and how does it relate to vitamin consumption? _____

    _____

7. What is a unit of measurement for vitamin A other than the microgram? _____

8. What nutrient can be produced by the body through exposure to sunshine? _____

9. Intestinal bacteria can produce what useful vitamin? _____

10. Name the eight B vitamins. _____

    _____

11. What is a coenzyme and what does it do? _____

    _____

12. What causes scurvy? _____

13. What are the benefits of phytochemicals, and how can you realize these benefits? _____

    _____

Interpret Implications

14. Explain the relationship between antioxidants and free radicals. What vitamins are antioxidants? _____

    _____

    _____

15. A dietitian works for a program for recovering alcoholics. What vitamin deficiency do you think the dietitian is most likely to encounter among her clients and why? _____

    _____

(Continued)

Name_____

16. Why do health experts recommend females increase their daily intake of folate between puberty and menopause? _____

_____

17. In most cases, do doctors advise getting vitamins from food items or from vitamin supplements? Explain.

_____

18. List four ways foods can lose vitamins. For each way listed, suggest a way this vitamin loss can be prevented.

_____

_____

_____

_____

_____

Apply & Practice

19. Write five personal goals you could set to help you meet all your vitamin needs.

_____

_____

_____

_____

_____

20. A flyer is being distributed outside a health foods store. The flyer promotes the sale of a vitamin E product by making the following claims:

Vitamin E... An Answer for Every Ailment...

E+
- *Maintains youthful vim, vigor, and vitality*
- *Maintains a healthy immune system*
- *Sustains peak performance*
- *Prevents tissue damage*
- *Protects blood cells*

Which claims are valid?

_____

Which are invalid?

_____

Minerals: Regulators of Body Functions

9

Mineral Match

Activity A

Chapter 9

Name _____

Date _____ Period _____

Match the following terms and identifying phrases.

_____ 1. An inorganic element needed in small amounts as a nutrient to perform various functions in the body.

_____ 2. Mineral required in the diet in an amount of 100 or more milligrams per day.

_____ 3. Mineral required in the diet in an amount of less than 100 milligrams per day.

_____ 4. A condition in which bones become porous and fragile due to a loss of minerals.

_____ 5. The time in a woman's life when menstruation ends due to a decrease in production of the hormone estrogen.

_____ 6. An abnormal cessation of menstrual periods.

_____ 7. The movement of water across a semipermeable membrane to equalize the concentrations of solution on each side of the membrane.

_____ 8. A compound that has a pH lower than 7.

_____ 9. A term used to express a substance's acidity or alkalinity.

_____ 10. An iron-containing protein that helps red blood cells carry oxygen from the lungs to cells throughout the body and carbon dioxide from body tissues back to the lungs for excretion.

_____ 11. A condition in which the number of red blood cells decline, causing the blood to have a decreased ability to carry oxygen to body tissues.

_____ 12. A substance that acts with enzymes to increase enzyme activity.

_____ 13. A hormone produced by the thyroid gland that helps control metabolism.

_____ 14. An enlargement of the thyroid gland.

_____ 15. Severe mental retardation and dwarfed physical features of an infant caused by the mother's iodine deficiency during pregnancy.

_____ 16. A spotty discoloration of teeth caused by high fluoride intake.

A. acid
B. amenorrhea
C. base
D. cofactor
E. cretinism
F. fluorosis
G. goiter
H. hemoglobin
I. iron-deficiency anemia
J. macromineral
K. menopause
L. micromineral
M. mineral
N. myoglobin
O. osmosis
P. osteoporosis
Q. pH
R. thyroxine

Go to the Source

Activity B   Name _____

Chapter 9   Date_____ Period _____

Complete the following chart by listing functions and food sources of each of the listed minerals. Then answer the question at the bottom of the page.

Minerals	Functions	Sources
Calcium		
Phosphorus		
Magnesium		
Sulfur		
Sodium		
Potassium		
Chloride		
Iron		
Zinc		
Iodine		
Fluoride		
Selenium		
Copper		
Chromium		
Manganese		
Molybdenum		

Do you eat food sources of each of the above minerals every day?_____

If not, which minerals may be lacking in your diet? _____

_____

Mineral Mysteries

Activity C   Name _____

Chapter 9   Date_____ Period _____

Choose the best response to complete each statement about mineral deficiencies and excesses. Write the letter in the space provided.

_____ 1. A gradual loss of bone density can result from a deficiency of _____.

    A. calcium   B. magnesium   C. phosphorus   D. sulfur

_____ 2. A great excess of _____ in the diet can cause fluorosis.

    A. chloride   B. fluoride   C. potassium   D. sodium

_____ 3. Deficiencies of _____ can result in anemia.

    A. copper   B. fluoride   C. iodine   D. zinc

_____ 4. Excessive amounts of _____ can cause liver damage, infections, and bloody stools.

    A. copper   B. chromium   C. iron   D. selenium

_____ 5. For people who are sensitive to this mineral, excess _____ can provoke hypertension.

    A. calcium   B. manganese   C. molybdenum   D. sodium

_____ 6. Goiter may be the result of a(n) _____ deficiency.

    A. magnesium   B. iodine   C. iron   D. phosphorus

_____ 7. Heart malfunctions can be a symptom of _____ deficiency.

    A. chloride   B. potassium   C. sodium   D. sulfur

_____ 8. Impaired glucose metabolism may be caused by a deficiency of _____.

    A. calcium   B. chloride   C. chromium   D. copper

_____ 9. Nausea, hair loss, and nerve damage are symptoms associated with an excess of _____.

    A. selenium   B. sodium   C. sulfur   D. zinc

_____ 10. Poor calcium absorption can be caused by excess _____ in the diet.

    A. fluoride   B. iodine   C. phosphorus   D. potassium

_____ 11. The most common type of anemia is caused by a deficiency of _____.

    A. copper   B. iodine   C. iron   D. selenium

_____ 12. Weakness, heart irregularities, disorientation, and seizures may result from a low intake of _____.

    A. calcium   B. magnesium   C. manganese   D. molybdenum

Minerals, More or Less

Activity D

Chapter 9

Name _____

Date_____ Period _____

Fill in the blank in each statement with either the word *more* or the word *less*.

1. Studying about mineral sources and functions can help people make _____ healthful decisions about foods.

2. Crops grown in soil that lacks minerals will contain _____ minerals than crops grown in mineral-rich soil.

3. _____ minerals are located in the outer layers of grain than in the inner parts.

4. _____ minerals are found near the peel of a fruit than in the center.

5. Plant foods provide _____ concentrated sources of minerals than animal foods.

6. Strict vegetarians may have a _____ mineral-rich diet than people who eat foods from animal sources.

7. Processed foods often have _____ mineral value than whole foods.

8. Fresh fruits and vegetables, whole grains, meat, poultry, and dairy products have _____ mineral value than fats, sugars, and refined flour.

9. Most adults absorb _____ than half of the minerals consumed in their diets.

10. Getting _____ minerals than the body requires can interfere with the absorption of other minerals.

11. Problems caused by mineral excesses are _____ often due to the use of supplements than food sources.

12. A diet that is too high in fiber can result in _____ mineral absorption.

13. The use of caffeine and other diuretics results in _____ urine output, thereby increasing the loss of minerals through excretion.

14. The body can absorb _____ calcium and phosphorus in the presence of vitamin D.

15. Eating foods high in vitamin C can result in _____ absorption of iron.

16. The body becomes _____ able to absorb many minerals during times of increased need.

17. Vitamins are _____ stable than minerals.

18. Vegetables that are soaked have _____ mineral content than those that are washed quickly.

19. Cooking methods that require little water promote _____ mineral retention than methods that require a lot of water.

20. Dishes made with the cooking liquid have _____ minerals than those where the cooking liquid is discarded.

Backtrack
Through Chapter 9

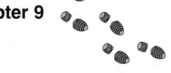

Activity E

Chapter 9

Name _____

Date_____ Period _____

Provide complete answers to the following questions and statements about minerals.

Recall the Facts

1. What is another name for macrominerals and how much of these minerals are needed in the diet? _____
   _____

2. List three functions of calcium other than building strong bones and teeth._____
   _____
   _____

3. Other than middle-aged women, what group of people is at risk of bone losses due to hormonal changes?
   _____

4. Why is excess phosphorus a problem? _____
   _____

5. A. Name three results of prolonged magnesium deficiency._____
   _____

   B. Name two results of severe magnesium toxicity.   _____
   _____

6. What mineral is found in high concentrations in hair, nails, and skin and produces a distinctive odor when burned?
   _____

7. What three minerals help regulate the fluid balance inside and outside the body cells? _____
   _____

8. List three symptoms of potassium deficiency._____
   _____

9. What are the two forms of iron and which is more easily absorbed?_____
   _____

10. At what times is adequate zinc intake most important? _____
    _____

11. What does an enlarged thyroid gland indicate? _____
    _____

12. What can be the result of a selenium deficiency? _____

(Continued)

Name_____

Interpret Implications

13. What are three problems that are more likely to be experienced by aging people who had inadequate calcium intake during their youth? _____

_____

14. How do sodium and potassium help maintain the proper pH of body fluids?_____

_____

15. Why do females ages 14 through 50 need more iron than males? _____

_____

16. How can excess zinc in the diet affect the body's use of other minerals? _____

_____

17. How can fluoridated drinking water affect the health of a community? _____

_____

_____

Apply & Practice

18. Your father has been diagnosed with hypertension. His doctor has advised him to reduce the sodium in his diet. Your whole family has agreed to modify their sodium intake to help support your father. How would you go about reducing the sodium in your diet? _____

_____

_____

19. You have been experiencing muscle cramps, loss of appetite, and constipation. What do you suspect the problem might be?_____

What would you do about it? _____

_____

_____

20. What are five steps you can take to be sure you are eating a mineral-rich diet?_____

_____

_____

_____

_____

Water: The Forgotten Nutrient

10

Water Crossword

Activity A

Chapter 10

Name _____

Date_____ Period _____

Across

2. A liquid in which substances can be dissolved is a _____.
5. Water outside the cells is _____cellular. (prefix)
8. This contains water to help lubricate food as you swallow it.
10. Water serves as a medium for _____ reactions.
12. A substance that reduces friction between surfaces is a _____.
15. A person who has an abnormal loss of body fluids is said to be _____.
17. A substance that increases urine production is a _____.
19. Water inside the cells is called _____cellular. (prefix)

Down

1. Regularly drinking excessive amounts of water can lead to water _____.
3. Body fluids that contain water are saliva, blood, digestive juices, urine, perspiration, and _____.
4. Water helps remove body wastes through exhaled water vapor, urine, feces, and _____.
6. This body tissue is about 75 percent water.
7. This body tissue is 20 to 35 percent water.
9. This is a lubricant for your eyes.
11. Body fluids that regulate body temperature are perspiration and _____.
13. Water is a _____product of nutrient metabolism. (prefix)
14. Kidneys form this when they draw water and wastes from the blood.
16. Most people need 2 to 3 _____ of water each day to replace body fluids.
18. Water determines the shape, size, and firmness of _____.

Drinking Water—The Undiluted Truth

Activity B   Name _____

Chapter 10   Date_____ Period _____

For each statement, write *T* in the blank if the statement is true or *F* in the blank if the statement is false. Then answer the questions at the bottom of the page.

_____ 1. The more expensive bottled waters are better for you than tap water.

_____ 2. Tap water often contains minerals that affect its taste.

_____ 3. Water from private wells may contain microorganisms.

_____ 4. Bottled water contains minerals that enhance your health.

_____ 5. Public water sources are tested and required to meet federal health standards.

_____ 6. Bottled water must meet higher standards for purity than public drinking water.

_____ 7. Private well water can be tested for contaminants.

_____ 8. Bottled water is always safer than tap water.

_____ 9. The presence of iron and sulfur deposits in water causes it to be hazardous.

_____10. The purity of tap water depends on the geographic location of the well.

Think It Over…

11. Do you prefer bottled water, filtered water, or tap water? Explain. _____

_____

_____

12. Why do you think bottled water is so popular? _____

_____

_____

13. Why do you think many people use filtration pitchers or systems? _____

_____

_____

14. Is bottled water worth the cost? Why or why not? _____

_____

_____

15. Are water filtration pitchers and systems worth the cost? Why or why not?_____

_____

Examining Your Water Needs

Activity C

Chapter 10

Name _____

Date_____ Period _____

Use this beverage diary to record your fluid consumption for 24 hours. (Remember to record your amounts in ounces.) Use Appendix B in the text to find the percentage of each beverage that is water. List this percentage in the third column. Next, for each beverage, find the ounces of water by multiplying the amount consumed by the percentage of water. Record this amount in the fourth column. Then, find the total ounces of water consumed by adding the ounces of water in each beverage. Write this number in the total box. Finally, answer the questions at the bottom of the page.

Beverage	Amount (oz.)	Percent Water	Ounces Water
		Total (oz.)	

1. How did the total ounces of water you consumed compare to the daily recommendation of 48 to 64 oz. (six to eight 8-ounce servings)?_____
_____

2. Foods contribute part of the body's needed water. Fruits and vegetables provide higher water contents than most other foods. Name four foods with a high water content you ate on the day of this beverage diary.____
_____
_____

3. Describe your activity level on the day of this beverage diary. _____
_____
_____

4. How does an increased activity level affect water needs? _____
_____

5. Write three goals that will help you improve your water consumption._____
_____
_____
_____

"Water Under the Bridge"

Activity D   **Name** _____

Chapter 10   **Date**_____ **Period** _____

You may have heard people use the expression "water under the bridge" when talking about past experiences. This implies that since the experience is in the past, it is best to forget it. Another way to look at past events is as learning experiences. Read the following mini-cases. In the spaces provided, tell what the teen in each case could learn to avoid similar situations in the future.

Case Situation 1

Sharon had been working in her grandmother's garden for over an hour. She was thirsty, so she quickly drank a quart of ice water from the thermos her grandfather brought. Sharon soon developed a pounding headache. She had to go inside and lie down.

_____

_____

_____

Case Situation 2

When he was sick with the flu, Sean went all day without eating or drinking. He had no appetite and very little thirst. By the end of the day, he was extremely weak and his fever had increased. When his father called the doctor, the first advice he received was to give Sean plenty of fluids.

_____

_____

_____

Case Situation 3

Harold was a member of the school wrestling team. During the summer he gained five pounds. He had just one week to lose the added weight before the new season began. He decided to fast, exercise, and take diuretics in order to reduce his water weight as quickly as possible.

_____

_____

_____

Case Situation 4

When she first started her running routine, Helen noticed she was always thirsty. She did not like the taste of her tap water. Instead, she drank one soft drink after another to try to quench her thirst. No matter how many soft drinks she drank, she was still thirsty. Finally, she decided to buy gallon jugs of bottled water, which seemed to work better.

_____

_____

_____

Backtrack
Through Chapter 10

Activity E

Chapter 10

Name _____

Date _____ **Period** _____

Provide complete answers to the following questions and statements about water.

Recall the Facts

1. The body contains approximately how many gallons of water? _____

2. For most adults, what percentage of body weight is water? _____

3. What are the five vital functions of water? _____

   _____

   _____

4. Give an example to illustrate that some foods are higher in water content than some beverages. _____

   _____

5. State three reasons some people buy bottled water instead of drinking tap water. _____

   _____

   _____

6. What is the average amount of water loss per person each day? _____

7. What are the four paths by which water leaves the body? _____

   _____

8. What is an electrolyte and what does it do? _____

   _____

9. What does a diuretic do? Give two examples of diuretics. _____

   _____

10. Why is it dangerous to lose 10 percent or more of your body weight through water losses? _____

    _____

11. How many 8-oz. glasses of liquids should a person drink each day? _____

12. What is considered to be a healthy urine output?_____

Interpret Implications

13. Explain why water is sometimes considered the most essential nutrient. _____

    _____

    _____

14. What does water do in its important role as a solvent? _____

    _____

    _____

(Continued)

Name_____

15. Explain how water helps regulate body temperature in both cold and warm weather conditions. _____
    _____
    _____

16. Explain how the water balance inside and outside the cells remains fairly constant. _____
    _____
    _____

17. Why do pregnant and lactating women have increased water needs?_____
    _____
    _____

Apply & Practice

18. Your doctor has advised you to increase your water intake. Which beverages would you choose to help you meet this goal and which would you avoid? Explain. _____
    _____
    _____
    _____
    _____

19. You have become ill with a stomach virus, which has left you unable to eat. Your doctor tells you it is okay to wait until you feel hungry before you eat again. The doctor says you should continue to drink plenty of fluids even if you are not thirsty. Is this good advice? Why or why not?_____
    _____
    _____
    _____
    _____

20. Name four specific ways you can include more water in your diet. _____
    _____
    _____
    _____

Nutrition for All Ages

The Life Cycle

Activity A

Chapter 11

Name _____

Date_____ Period _____

For each numbered segment of the life cycle diagram below, write the name of that stage in the corresponding blank to the right. For each stage, indicate the ages when a person enters and exits that stage. Then answer the questions at the bottom of the page.

Life Cycle Diagram

1. Stage: _____
   Ages: _____
2. Stage: _____
   Ages: _____
3. Stage: _____
   Ages: _____
4. Stage: _____
   Ages: _____
5. Stage: _____
   Ages: _____

6. Using your own words, define *life cycle*. _____
_____

7. Explain why nutrition experts subdivide some stages of the life cycle into more specific life-stage groups.
_____

8. Give the age ranges for the two life-stage groups within adolescence. _____

   On the life cycle diagram, draw a line to indicate the division between these two life-stage groups. Shade in the life-stage group to which you belong.

9. What happens to nutrient needs for adults? _____
_____

   Give the age ranges for the four life-stage groups within adulthood. _____
_____

   On the life cycle diagram, draw lines to indicate the divisions between these life-stage groups.

10. Explain why it is important to understand the life cycle when considering nutritional needs. _____
_____
_____

Nutrition During Pregnancy

Activity B

Chapter 11

Name _____

Date_____ Period _____

Complete the following statements about changing nutritional needs during pregnancy.

_____ 1. A name for producing breast milk is _____.

_____ 2. Care that is given during a woman's pregnancy to reduce the risk of complications to both mother and fetus is called _____.

_____ 3. Women who become pregnant when they are 10 percent or more below healthy weight have a greater risk of having a _____ baby, or a baby that is too small.

_____ 4. A _____ baby is one that is born before the 35th week of pregnancy.

_____ 5. Each one-third of pregnancy (about 13 to 14 weeks) is called a _____.

_____ 6. Pregnant women need to consume extra _____ to build fetal tissue and support changes in their own bodies. Many already get more than enough of this nutrient.

_____ 7. An increased amount of the vitamin _____ is needed to aid in the development of the baby's brain and spinal cord.

_____ 8. Pregnant women who are vegetarians need to eat fortified foods or take supplements containing vitamin _____. This vitamin occurs naturally only in animal foods.

_____ 9. Pregnant women must consume enough _____ to prevent losses from their bones.

_____ 10. Four minerals besides calcium for which a woman's needs increase during pregnancy are _____.

_____

_____

_____

_____ 11. Along with extra nutrients, pregnant women need additional _____ from the food they eat to supply energy to support fetal development.

_____ 12. Average weight gain during pregnancy for a woman of normal weight is between _____ and _____ pounds.

_____ 13. Pregnant women should limit foods that are high in _____ and low in other nutrients.

_____ 14. Nausea that often occurs during pregnancy is called _____.

_____ 15. In pregnant women, _____ has been linked to having low-birthweight babies. It causes babies to be deprived of oxygen, which endangers their health.

_____ 16. Any substances in the mother's blood pass into the bloodstream of the fetus through the blood vessels in the _____.

_____ 17. During pregnancy, the use of legal or illegal drugs increases the risk of _____ disabilities in the fetus.

_____ 18. _____ is a set of disorders that includes brain damage, retarded growth, and irregular facial features. It is often present in infants whose mothers drank alcohol during pregnancy.

Feeding an Infant

Activity C   Name _____

Chapter 11   Date_____ Period _____

Complete the following activities related to infant feeding.

Complete the following statements about feeding schedules for infants.

1. Most babies require _____ feedings per day.

2. After the first few weeks, caregivers can space feedings for babies at _____ hour intervals.

3. At _____ months, feedings can decrease to five a day.

4. At _____ months, feedings can decrease to four a day.

Rank each of the following foods in the order it is mostly likely to be introduced in an infant's diet. Start with 1 for the first food.

_____5. cereals   _____8. apple juice

_____6. strained fruits   _____9. meats

_____7. breast milk or iron-   _____10. strained vegetables
         fortified formula

Complete the following sentences about tips for feeding infants.

11. Introducing one food at a time helps caregivers identify _____.

12. Caregivers should avoid overfeeding infants to prevent _____.

13. Holding foods with their hands helps prepare infants to _____.

14. Infants need frequent feedings because _____.

15. When a baby rejects a food, he or she is showing

    _____.

16. When a caregiver acts negatively toward a food, a child may learn to

    _____.

Sticky Situations

Activity D

Chapter 11

Name _____

Date_____ Period _____

A number of eating problems can arise when children reach the toddler stage. Read these "sticky situations" and answer the questions that follow.

1. Fifteen-month-old Sarah ate a few bites of her spaghetti. Then she smeared the sauce on the tray of the high chair and threw the noodles on the floor.

   A. Why do you think Sarah is such a messy eater? _____

   _____

   _____

   B. What advice would you give her caregiver? _____

   _____

   _____

2. One-year-old Theodore choked twice during his lunch of beanie weanies and a sliced banana.

   A. Why might this meal have caused Theodore to choke? _____

   _____

   _____

   B. What advice would you give his caregiver? _____

   _____

   _____

3. Eighteen-month-old Ronald usually eats his lunch in front of the TV while his mom watches her favorite show. Ronald usually eats very little before getting down to play.

   A. Why do you think Ronald eats so little? _____

   _____

   _____

   B. What advice would you give his mother? _____

   _____

   _____

4. Two-year-old Cathy is usually a good eater. Recently she has not wanted to eat her food. She has rejected even her favorites. Cathy's caregiver doesn't know what to do.

   A. What are some reasons why Cathy may have become a picky eater? _____

   _____

   _____

   B. What advice would you give her caregiver? _____

   _____

   _____

Ticket to Teen Nutrition

Activity E   Name _____

Chapter 11   Date _____ Period _____

Fill in the blanks to complete these statements about teen nutrition.

1. _____ is the period of life between childhood and adulthood.

2. _____ is the time during which a person reaches sexual maturity.

3. Most adolescents experience a period of rapid physical growth that is known as a _____.

4. Body _____ changes during adolescence as females develop a layer of fatty tissue and males develop more lean body mass.

5. A teen's daily calorie needs are _____ than they were in late childhood.

6. The average teen female needs _____ calories per day.

7. Teen males need more calories than teen females because they have more _____.

8. An 18-year-old male needs _____ more calories per day than when he was 13 years old.

9. Teens need to replenish supplies of energy and nutrients at _____ intervals throughout the day.

10. _____ eating patterns can cause teens to be tired, irritable, drowsy, and distracted.

11. Breakfast should provide _____ of a teen's daily nutrient needs.

12. Teens should choose fast foods in _____ because they are high in sugar, fat, and sodium.

13. Some teens who do not consume enough iron may develop _____.

14. Females need more iron than males due to _____.

15. Weight problems of teens include overweight, underweight, and eating _____.

16. Inadequate calcium intake during the teen years can affect bone _____.

17. Too much sugar during the teen years can cause dental _____.

18. A high-fat diet during the teen years can increase the risk of _____ disease in later life.

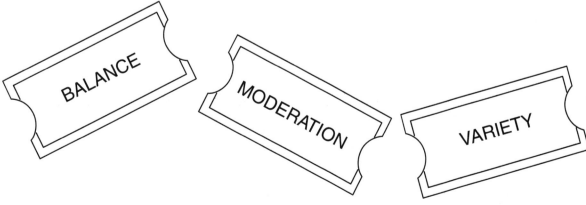

Advice for Adults

Activity F   **Name** _____

Chapter 11   **Date** _____ **Period** _____

Read the case situations involving adult nutrition advice. In the space provided, explain whether the advice given was good or bad and explain why. For any instances of bad advice, offer a better suggestion.

1. Mary tells her doctor she does not like milk and has always avoided dairy products to help keep her weight down. The doctor advises her to begin taking a calcium supplement before she approaches the age of menopause.

    _____

    _____

    _____

2. Jenny's mother is 75 years old and lives alone in the country. Lately, she has been eating very little and losing weight. She says she has no appetite. A friend advised Jenny to bring her mother home for the weekend and try to make her eat before things get worse.

    _____

    _____

    _____

3. Pat notices her husband has been gaining weight in the past few weeks. His pants are too tight in the waist, and he is using new holes in his belts. She advises him to pay more attention to what he is eating. She reminds her husband it's better to keep weight off than to try to lose it later.

    _____

    _____

    _____

4. George has been having problems with constipation. He mentioned this to his brother, who advised him to eat a high-fiber diet and drink lots of fluids.

    _____

    _____

    _____

5. Since his wife died, Bob has had to cook his own meals. He has found cooking for one to be challenging. His daughter asked him to try lunches offered at the Sunny Senior Center.

    _____

    _____

    _____

Backtrack
Through Chapter 11

Activity G

Chapter 11

Name _____

Date_____ Period _____

Provide complete answers to the following questions and statements about nutrition throughout the life cycle.

Recall the Facts

1. Which stages of the life cycle have you already completed? _____

2. How does gender determine the amounts of nutrients a person needs?_____

3. Why do a woman's nutritional needs change during pregnancy?_____

4. When a mother chooses to breast-feed, what nutrients does she need in even greater amounts than when she was pregnant? _____

5. What harmful effects can FAS have on a baby?_____

6. During what stage is growth more rapid than at any other stage? _____

7. What is generally considered to be the ideal food for infants and why?_____

8. Give an example of a toddler-sized serving for a food from the grains group.

9. The childhood stage of the life cycle includes which ages? _____

10. List four healthful snacks parents can provide for children. _____

11. What are two major causes of childhood weight problems?_____

12. How does a growth spurt affect nutritional needs?_____

13. List the names and age ranges of the four stages into which nutrition experts divide adulthood. _____

(Continued)

Name_____

Interpret Implications

14. Why is it important to understand the life cycle when considering a person's nutritional needs? _____
_____
_____

15. How can drugs used by a mother harm her baby during pregnancy and lactation? _____
_____

16. Describe how teen pregnancy causes special problems not seen in the pregnancies of adult women. _____
_____
_____

17. How can healthful eating increase a person's ability to perform well in school or on the job?_____
_____

18. Briefly describe three ways nutritional needs change after age 50. _____
_____
_____

Apply & Practice

19. Plan a day's menus for a teen using the nutritional information from the chapter.

Breakfast	Lunch	Snack	Dinner

20. List two tips to consider when planning meals for someone in each of the following stages of the life cycle.

A. infancy_____
_____

B. toddlerhood _____
_____

C. childhood_____
_____

D. adolescence _____
_____

E. adulthood _____
_____

The Energy Balancing Act

In Balance

Activity A

Name _____

Chapter 12

Date_____ Period _____

Use the clues provided to identify terms related to energy balance. Write one letter in each space. Use the circled letters to name the two sides of the energy balance equation at the bottom of the page.

1. The concentration of energy in a food is referred to as __ __ __ __ __ __ __   __(__)__ __ __ __.

2. An adult with a body mass index below 18.5 is defined as __(__)__ __ __ __ __ __ __ __ __.

3. The energy required to complete the processes of digestion, absorption, and metabolism is called the __ __ __ __ __ __ __ __(__)__ __ __ __ __   __ __   __ __ __ __.

4. The rate at which the body uses energy for basal metabolism is called the __ __ __ __ __ __ __ __ __ __ __ __ __ __(__)__ __ __.

5. __ __ __ __(__)__ is the ability to do work.

6. A __ __ __ __ __ __ __(__)   __ __ __ __ __ __ __ __ is an activity that requires a lot of sitting.

7. The amount of energy required to support the operation of all internal body systems except digestion is known as __ __ __ __ __   __ __ __ __ __ __ __(__)__ __.

8. A process that measures body fat by measuring the body's resistance to a low-energy electrical current is __ __ __ __ __ __ __ __ __ __ __ __ __   __ __ __ __ __ __(__)__ __.

9. Compounds formed from fatty acids the nervous system can use for energy when carbohydrates are not available are called __ __ __ __ __(__)   __ __ __ __ __ __ __.

10. A test in which the thickness of a fold of skin is measured to estimate the amount of subcutaneous fat is called a __ __ __(__)__ __ __ __   __ __ __ __.

11. An adult with a body mass index of 30 or more is defined as __ __(__)__ __.

12. An adult with a body mass index of 25 to 29.9 is defined as __ __ __(__)__ __ __ __ __.

13. An adult with a body mass index of 18.5 to 24.9 is defined as having __ __ __ __ __ __ __   __ __ __(__)__ __.

14. A calculation of body weight and height used to define underweight, healthy weight, overweight, and obesity is __ __ __(__)   __ __ __ __ __   __ __ __ __ __.

15. The percentage of different types of tissues in the body, such as fat, muscle, and bone, refers to __ __ __ __ __ __ __ __(__)__ __ __ __ __.

16. Fat that lies underneath the skin is called __ __ __ __(__)__ __ __ __ __ __ __   __ __ __.

17. An abnormal buildup of ketone bodies in the bloodstream is a condition known as __ __(__)__ __ __ __.

The Energy Balance Equation

__ __ __ __ __ __   __ __   =   __ __ __ __ __ __ __   __ __ __

Calorie Calculations

Activity B

Chapter 12

Name _____

Date_____ Period _____

Show the calculations you use to solve each of the following problems involving energy input and output.

1. The Nutrition Facts panel on a box of macaroni and cheese tells you a serving provides 230 calories. The panel shows a serving provides 90 calories from fat. A serving provides 9 grams of protein and 26 grams of carbohydrate. How many calories come from protein and carbohydrate?

2. Your physician advises you to limit your fat intake to no more than 30 percent of your daily calories. Suppose your daily diet included 260 grams of carbohydrates, 75 grams of fat, and 60 grams of protein. Are you following your doctor's advice? Explain.

3. A broiled chicken sandwich weighs 248 grams and provides 540 calories. A double bacon cheeseburger weighs 159 grams and provides 460 calories. Which of the two fast foods is more calorie dense?

4. What would be the basal energy needs per day of a man who weighs 175 pounds?

5. Refer to Chart 12-6 on page 216 in the text. Use the average in each range of calories. Estimate the number of calories Carlos burned through physical activity from 7:00 AM to 12:00 noon on Saturday morning. Carlos rose at 7:00 for an early morning run. He returned at 8:00, had breakfast, and read the paper until 9:00. Then he showered, dressed, washed dishes, and cleaned the kitchen until 10:00. From 10:00 to noon, he raked leaves.

6. Stephanie burns about 2,400 calories per day. Approximately how many of these calories are for each of the following needs: basal metabolism, physical activity, and thermic effect of food?

Health Hangs in the Balance

Activity C

Chapter 12

Name _____

Date_____ Period _____

Read the following statements about energy imbalance. Circle *T* if the statement is true. Circle *F* if the statement is false.

T F 1. Going on a weight-loss diet is an example of creating an intentional energy deficiency.

T F 2. Energy deficiency occurs when energy output is less than energy intake.

T F 3. Energy deficiencies may be caused by poverty, famine, illness, or dieting.

T F 4. When there is an energy deficiency, the body draws first on fatty tissue to meet its needs.

T F 5. The stored form of glucose from carbohydrates for use by nonmuscle tissue is liver glycogen.

T F 6. Glycogen stores will be depleted within two to three hours after the body begins to draw on them for energy.

T F 7. Weight loss occurs as the body draws on fatty tissue for energy.

T F 8. The nervous system uses only fat as a fuel source.

T F 9. The body can convert fat into glucose for use as a fuel source.

T F 10. The body can easily make glucose from amino acids to feed the nervous system without any health consequences.

T F 11. Breaking down muscle proteins causes a rapid weight loss due to loss of body fluids.

T F 12. Changing fatty acids into ketone bodies is the body's way of limiting muscle deterioration when carbohydrates are not available.

T F 13. A buildup of ketone bodies in the bloodstream is a sign of good health.

T F 14. Ketosis changes the acid-base balance of the blood.

T F 15. Low-carbohydrate diets are recommended by most nutritionists.

T F 16. A weight-loss diet needs to include adequate amounts of carbohydrates to prevent damage to body protein tissues.

T F 17. Energy excess occurs when energy output is less than energy intake.

T F 18. Excess calories are stored as adipose tissue.

T F 19. An excess of 2,400 calories in the diet leads to one pound of stored body fat.

T F 20. The amount of weight a person gains within a given time depends on the degree of energy excess.

T F 21. Just a small daily energy excess can result in a number of added pounds of body fat over a period of years.

T F 22. The more excess fat a body has, the greater the risks for health problems.

Evaluate Your Weight

Activity D   Name _____

Chapter 12   Date_____ Period _____

Complete the following exercises to help you evaluate your weight and compare various weight evaluation tools.

1. What is your height in inches? _____

2. What is your weight in pounds? _____

Body Mass Index

3. Calculate your body mass index by completing the following equations.

   A. _____ × _____ = _____
      height   height   height^2

   B. _____ ÷ _____ = _____
      weight   height^2 X

   C. _____ × 705 = _____
      X   constant   BMI

4. What does your BMI indicate about the status of your weight? _____

   _____

5. Do you think body mass index is an appropriate weight evaluation tool for you? _____

   Explain why or why not. _____

   _____

Height-Weight Tables

6. What is the healthy weight range shown in a height-weight table for someone of your height? _____

7. Where does your weight fall in relation to this range? _____

   _____

8. What does this indicate about your weight? _____

   _____

9. Are height-weight tables an appropriate weight evaluation tool for you? _____

   Explain why or why not. _____

   _____

Body Fat Measurement

10. Do a pinch test by grasping the skin on the back of your upper arm halfway between your shoulder and elbow. Pinch this fold of skin between your thumb and forefinger. Be sure to grasp only the fat, not the muscle. What is the distance between your thumb and forefinger? _____

11. What does this indicate about your weight? _____

    _____

12. Is the pinch test an appropriate weight evaluation tool for you?_____

    Explain why or why not. _____

Backtrack
Through Chapter 12

Activity E

Chapter 12

Name _____

Date _____ Period _____

Provide complete answers to the following questions and statements about energy balance.

Recall the Facts

1. What type of energy is stored in food? _____

2. From what three nutrient groups does the body obtain food energy? _____

   _____

3. What three factors account for the calories you expend each day? _____

   _____

4. Which internal body system is not included in the amount of energy designated for basal metabolism? ____

   _____

5. What hormone regulates basal metabolism? _____

6. What three aspects of physical activity cause an increase in energy needs? _____

   _____

7. Name five activities that would be described as sedentary. _____

   _____

8. What term refers to the energy required to get the energy from food? _____

9. What is the first step the body takes to meet its energy needs when there is not enough food energy available?

   _____

10. Without stating a BMI range, describe what it means to have a healthy body weight._____

    _____

11. List one disadvantage of determining healthy weight using height-weight tables. _____

    _____

12. What percentage of fat in the body is subcutaneous fat?_____

Interpret Implications

13. Explain why foods that are high in water are low in calorie density and foods that are high in fats are high in calorie density._____

    _____

    _____

14. Why would a 150-pound member of the women's swim team burn more calories than her 110-pound team-mate swimming at the same pace?_____

    _____

(Continued)

Name_____

15. Why might someone intentionally create an energy imbalance in his or her body?_____

_____

16. How can a small daily energy excess affect health? _____

_____

17. Explain why the location of body fat appears to affect health. _____

_____

_____

Apply & Practice

18. Use the Recommended Dietary Allowances chart in Appendix A to find your recommended energy intake. How does that amount compare with your recommended intake ten years ago, five years ago, five years from now, and ten years from now? Why do you think the amounts change? _____

_____

_____

_____

_____

19. Explain what factors might cause your BMR to differ from that of an inactive; five-foot, two-inch; 50-year-old woman.

_____

_____

_____

_____

20. Mrs. Swanson is five feet six inches tall, and she weighs 145 pounds. Her 16-year-old twins, Jake and Janet, are the same height and weight as their mother. What is the body mass index of these family members?

_____

What does this BMI indicate about each person's weight? Explain your answer. _____

_____

_____

_____

Healthy Weight Management

Weigh the Risks

Activity A

Chapter 13

Name _____

Date _____ Period _____

The list below contains health risks of being overweight and risks of being underweight. Each risk is identified by a letter. If a risk is associated with being underweight, write the letter in the pan of the scale labeled "underweight." If the risk is associated with being overweight, write the letter in the "overweight" pan. Note that some risks belong in both pans. Be prepared to support your answers. In the space provided, write a paragraph about the risk of most interest to you. Summarize ways to "tip the scales in your favor."

A. arthritis

B. cancer

C. coronary heart disease

D. diabetes

E. discrimination

F. eating disorders

G. fatigue

H. high blood pressure

I. inability to stay warm

J. inadequate nutrient stores

K. irregular menstruation

L. low self-esteem

M. pregnancy problems

N. respiratory problems

O. surgical problems

Scale

Summary

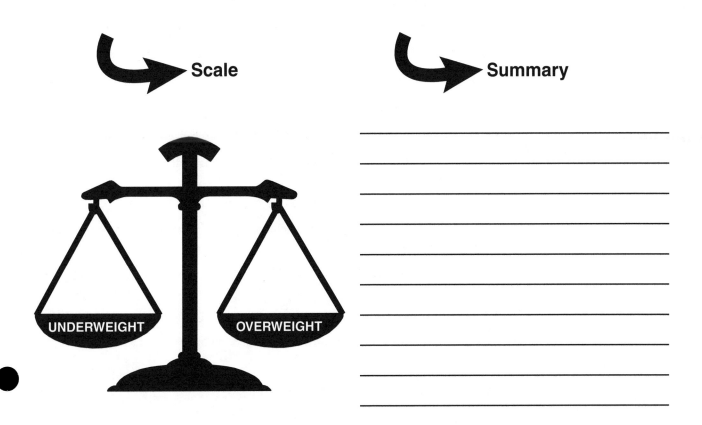

UNDERWEIGHT   OVERWEIGHT

Facts and Factors

Activity B   Name _____

Chapter 13   Date_____ Period _____

Examine the following statements about factors affecting weight status. If the statement is true, write *true* in the blank. If the statement is false, change the underlined word or phrase to make the statement true. Write the correct word or phrase in the blank.

_____ 1. Weight <u>management</u> means how much you weigh and your ability to gain or lose weight.

_____ 2. <u>Heredity</u> affects the shape of your body.

_____ 3. The size of your bones and the location of fat stores on the body are <u>inherited</u> traits.

_____ 4. Your <u>heredity</u> affects basal metabolic rate.

_____ 5. A family history of obesity <u>does</u> necessarily mean you will be obese, too.

_____ 6. Weight management may be <u>easier</u> for a person who inherited genes that lean toward obesity.

_____ 7. Parents <u>can</u> greatly influence a child's eating habits.

_____ 8. Parents can plan their children's meals and snacks around appropriate portions of <u>nutritious</u> foods.

_____ 9. Teens have <u>more</u> control over what they eat than children do.

_____10. Many teens form habits of eating foods that are <u>low</u> in fat and calories.

_____11. Eating habits <u>may</u> be influenced by schedules, peers, and weight concerns.

_____12. <u>Work and family</u> obligations sometimes negatively affect eating patterns.

_____13. Adults who commute to work often eat <u>at home</u>.

_____14. Situations that trigger you to eat are called environmental <u>cues</u>.

_____15. Social settings and time of day are examples of <u>hereditary</u> factors that influence weight status.

_____16. Being aware of when and why you eat <u>is not</u> important.

_____17. Examples of <u>environmental</u> factors include depression, boredom, fear, tension, and loneliness.

_____18. People <u>can</u> look for appropriate ways to deal with their emotions while following a nutritious diet.

_____19. Physical activity influences the "calories <u>in</u>" side of the energy balance equation.

_____20. An <u>active</u> lifestyle can lead to an energy excess and unwanted weight gain.

The Math of Weight Loss

Activity C   **Name** _____

Chapter 13   **Date**_____ **Period** _____

Read the following situations that require mathematical calculations related to weight loss. Use the formulas presented in this chapter to solve them. Show your work.

1. Henry is a very active teen who weighs 140 pounds. Approximately what are his daily energy needs in calories?

2. Two teens are arguing over which of them needs more calories each day. Serena is 15, lightly active, and weighs 125 pounds. Salena is 17, moderately active, and weighs 145 pounds. Who needs more calores per day?

3. Brandon has cut his caloric intake by 350 calories per day. How long will it take him to lose one pound?

4. Tom is a weight lifter on the high school team. His trainer advised him to lose three pounds in the next four weeks. How much is the daily calorie deficit he needs to create, either by reducing calorie intake or increasing calorie needs? Does that amount appear to be a safe goal?

5. Marlita kept a food log for a week. She learned she has been averaging 2,100 calories per day. She is 16, moderately active, and weighs 135 pounds. Is her intake greater than or less than her caloric needs? What advice would you offer?

Believe It or Not?

Activity D

Chapter 13

Name _____

Date_____ Period _____

A new weight loss center has just opened in town. Operators of the center claim to have the best and latest methods for weight loss. Evaluate each claim posted on the storefront below. In the space provided at the bottom of the page, write *believe it* next to the claims you believe and *not* next to the claims you do not believe. Write a brief statement to support each response.

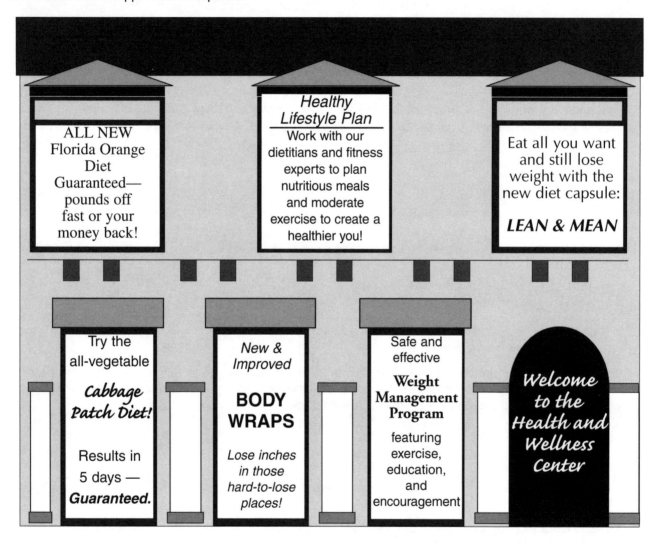

1. Florida Orange Diet

2. Healthy Lifestyle Plan

3. Lean & Mean

4. Cabbage Patch Diet

5. Body Wraps

6. Weight Management Program

In the Driver's Seat

Activity E

Chapter 13

Name _____

Date_____ Period _____

When it comes to weight management, it seems everyone has advice to give. Read each piece of advice below. In the blanks, write *GA* for each piece of good advice and *BA* for each piece of bad advice. Then in the space provided, explain why the advice is good or bad. When it comes to weight management, you are in the driver's seat—you are in control of your own food intake and energy balance.

_____ 1. Think of food as the enemy and self-denial as the goal.

   _____

_____ 2. See a doctor before you begin a weight loss program.

   _____

_____ 3. Think of losing weight as managing intake, not as dieting.

   _____

_____ 4. Read any weight loss plan you are considering carefully and thoroughly.

   _____

_____ 5. The best diets are those that allow you to take off pounds quickly.

   _____

_____ 6. Choose a diet that is as close to your food preferences as possible.

   _____

_____ 7. The all-carrot diet is a good choice because carrots have a lot of vitamins.

   _____

_____ 8. A good diet should allow you to eat out without social discomfort or embarrassment.

   _____

_____ 9. Avoid diets that are based on the use of pills.

   _____

_____10. Fasting is well-named because it is the fastest and best way to lose weight.

   _____

_____11. To lose weight, cut down on vegetables and whole-grain foods.

   _____

_____12. Lose weight slowly to avoid health risks.

   _____

_____13. Replace high-fat snacks with fresh fruits.

   _____

_____14. Keep a food diary to help identify problem eating behaviors.

   _____

_____15. Two or three square meals a day are better than five or six smaller meals.

   _____

_____16. A good way to cut calories is to skip breakfast.

   _____

_____17. Choose steamed or broiled, not fried, foods when you eat out.

   _____

(Continued)

Name_____

_____18. Drink a glass of water before a meal so you will not feel so hungry.

_____

_____19. Weigh yourself only once or twice a week.

_____

_____20. Always clean your plate.

_____

_____21. Consider going to see a registered dietitian to get counseling about weight loss.

_____

_____22. Diet pills are not addictive as long as you follow the recommended dosage.

_____

_____23. Substitute low-calorie ingredients in the recipes you prepare at home.

_____

_____24. Increase your physical activity to help curb short-term hunger.

_____

_____25. Use a smaller plate so your portions of food do not look so small.

_____

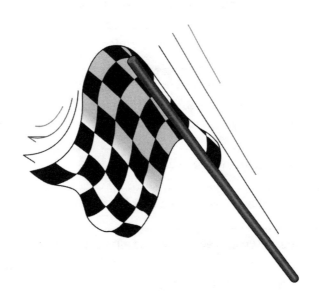

Backtrack
Through Chapter 13

Activity F

Chapter 13

Name _____

Date _____ Period _____

Provide complete answers to the following questions and statements about healthy weight management.

Recall the Facts
- -

1. What does weight management mean? _____
_____

2. What percentage of people in the United States are overweight or obese? _____

3. Why is reducing obesity a national health goal in the United States? _____

4. List three reasons being underweight can be a problem. _____
_____

5. List three types of factors that influence weight status. _____

6. Name three environmental cues that affect eating habits. _____
_____

7. What energy deficit in calories is needed to lose one pound of body fat? _____

8. What is the recommended range of calorie deficit per day? _____

9. Does a higher level of activity increase or decrease a person's daily calorie needs? _____

10. What is the difference between a fad diet and a crash diet? _____
_____

11. What is weight cycling? _____
_____

12. In general, how much weight can a person safely lose in one week? _____

13. If a person is trying to gain weight, why should he or she avoid drinking extra fluids just before mealtime?
_____

Interpret Implications
- -

14. List two disadvantages of liquid diet programs. _____
_____

15. What causes a person to gain weight? _____
_____
_____

(Continued)

Name_____

16. To what extent does the FDA protect consumers from false weight-loss claims? _____

_____

_____

17. What are the dangers of fasting? _____

_____

_____

18. Suggest five ways an underweight person might work toward safe weight gain. _____

_____

_____

_____

Apply & Practice

19. While being overweight is almost always seen as a health concern, being underweight is commonly over-looked as a health concern. Why do you think this is? What, if anything, can be done to change this? _____

_____

_____

_____

20. This chapter describes several ways to change eating habits—keeping a food diary, using activities to manage emotions, finding new responses to cues, writing a habit change contract, and setting up a points system. If your doctor advised you to lose or gain weight, which approach would work best for you and why?

_____

_____

_____

_____

_____

Eating Disorders

14

Read the Warning Signs

Name _____

Date _____ Period _____

Read the following list of characteristics and health risks associated with various eating disorders. If an item describes anorexia nervosa, write *AN* in the blank. If an item describes bulimia nervosa, write *BN* in the blank. If an item describes binge eating disorder, write *BED* in the blank. Some items may describe more than one eating disorder.

_____ 1. A cycle of bingeing and purging is repeated at least twice a week.

_____ 2. A sense of power is derived from controlling weight.

_____ 3. Amenorrhea develops among females.

_____ 4. Baggy clothes may be used to help hide an overly thin body.

_____ 5. Behavior is hidden from others.

_____ 6. Denial becomes an obstacle to treatment.

_____ 7. Dieting becomes a life-threatening obsession.

_____ 8. Eating patterns are recognized as abnormal.

_____ 9. Excessive exercise may be used to prevent weight gain.

_____ 10. Fear of weight gain is intense.

_____ 11. Feeling cold is a common complaint.

_____ 12. Feelings of guilt about overeating are common.

_____ 13. Forced vomiting may be used to prevent weight gain.

_____ 14. Health problems may result from excess weight.

_____ 15. Huge amounts of food are eaten uncontrollably.

_____ 16. No steps are taken to prevent weight gain.

_____ 17. Personality is highly achievement oriented.

_____ 18. Throat glands may become swollen.

_____ 19. Tooth enamel may be destroyed by stomach acids.

_____ 20. Weight-loss programs are often not completed.

Help for Eating Disorders

Activity B

Chapter 14

Name _____

Date_____ Period _____

In the space provided, briefly describe the role each of the following people may play in the treatment of eating disorders.

1. medical doctor

   _____
   _____
   _____

2. psychologist

   _____
   _____
   _____

3. registered dietitian

   _____
   _____
   _____

4. exercise specialist

   _____
   _____
   _____

5. family members

   _____
   _____
   _____

6. friends

   _____
   _____
   _____

7. support group members

   _____
   _____
   _____

8. family therapist

   _____
   _____
   _____

What role must a person with an eating disorder play in his or her treatment?

_____
_____
_____

Evaluating Theories

Activity C   **Name** _____

Chapter 14   **Date** _____ **Period** _____

Three main theories about the causes of eating disorders are described in the text. The first three parts of this activity focus on each of these theories. In the final part, write your conclusions about the causes of eating disorders.

Part One: Social Pressure Theory

This theory says social pressure to be thin prompts people to form unhealthful eating habits. Cut an example of an advertisement from a magazine or newspaper that uses this type of pressure. Staple the ad to this page. Then answer the following questions about your ad.

1. How does your ad create pressure to be thin? _____

    _____

    _____

2. Is the message direct or indirect? Explain. _____

    _____

3. Explain why this ad might be a greater influence on teens than on adults. _____

    _____

    _____

4. Do you think this ad might affect athletes more than nonathletes? Explain. _____

    _____

    _____

Part Two: Genetic Link Theory

Using library resources and/or the Internet, research the theory that eating disorders may have a genetic link. Then answer the following questions.

1. Names of resources used or Internet addresses visited: _____

    _____

    _____

2. How would you summarize any information you found about genetics and eating disorders? _____

    _____

    _____

3. When a person has an eating disorder, do you think most people suspect genetic influences as the cause? Explain. _____

    _____

    _____

4. Does your research indicate how, if at all, the genetic causes of eating disorders can be treated? Explain.

    _____

    _____

(Continued)

Name_____

Part Three: Family Pattern Theory

This theory suggests the interactions between family members may be related to the development of eating disorders. Use the following questions to interview a doctor or dietitian. Summarize the person's responses in the space provided.

1. What role do family relationships play in a person's eating disorder? _____

_____

_____

2. Are teens more vulnerable to family influences than people of other ages? Explain. _____

_____

_____

3. Why might family members have trouble identifying an eating disorder?_____

_____

_____

4. How can families change to support the recovery of a person with an eating disorder? _____

_____

_____

Part Four: Conclusions

Answer the following questions about your conclusions regarding theories concerning eating disorders.

1. With which theory do you most agree? Explain._____

_____

_____

_____

2. Is it possible for a person to agree with all three theories? Why or why not?_____

_____

3. Are the causes of eating disorders more complex than you had previously thought? Explain. _____

_____

_____

4. Can you identify other factors that cause eating disorders that are not addressed by these theories? If so, what are they?_____

_____

Backtrack
Through Chapter 14

Activity D
Chapter 14

Name _____

Date _____ Period _____

Provide complete answers to the following questions and statements about eating disorders.

Recall the Facts

1. What are the three most common eating disorders? _____

   _____

2. To what two groups of people are eating disorders most common? _____

3. What type of origin is denoted by the label *nervosa*? _____

   _____

4. Name four methods used by bulimics to purge. _____

   _____

5. What are three emotions that often accompany binge eating disorder? _____

   _____

6. Name one major source of social pressure to be thin. _____

7. What three types of family patterns have been associated with the development of eating disorders? _____

   _____

   _____

8. What three medical problems comprise the female athlete triad? _____

   _____

9. What are the chances that an anorexic will recover completely if given proper treatment? _____

   _____

10. What is outpatient treatment? _____

11. What is the goal of counseling in treating binge eating disorder? _____

    _____

12. What role would a registered dietitian play in treating someone with an eating disorder? _____

    _____

Interpret Implications

13. What motivates anorexics to keep dieting? _____

    _____

    _____

(Continued)

Name_____

14. Why are bulimics sometimes harder to identify than anorexics? _____
    _____

15. Why is the risk of developing an eating disorder higher during the teen years? _____
    _____

16. How can verbal skills and stress management techniques help someone who has anorexia nervosa? _____
    _____

17. How can recovering bulimics avoid having relapses?_____
    _____

Apply & Practice

18. Suppose you are a member of a sports team at school. The coach repeatedly tells team members they must
    watch their weight if they want to compete. What could you privately say to the coach about his or her
    influence on the development of eating disorders among team members? _____
    _____

    _____

19. How could you help a family member with an eating disorder feel comfortable with members of a health care
    team? _____
    _____

    _____

20. What would you do if you believed your friend was bulimic? _____
    _____

    _____

Staying Physically Active: A Way of Life

Assessing Activity Goals

Activity A

Chapter 15

Name _____

Date _____ **Period** _____

Provide honest answers to the following questions about your physical activity habits. Then determine which of the three main goals for physical activity you have—good health, total fitness, and/or peak athletic performance.

1. How much time do you spend each day engaged in moderate activity (such as walking, riding a bicycle, raking, and sweeping)? _____

_____

_____

2. What physical activities are part of your daily routine?_____

_____

_____

_____

3. What household tasks do you do regularly?_____

_____

_____

4. Do you participate in any regular exercise programs? If so, describe.

_____

_____

_____

5. Are you involved in any training programs to develop specific sports skills? Describe the programs and what skills you are developing.

_____

_____

6. What seem to be your main goals for physical activity? _____

_____

_____

7. Suggest three ways you can meet each main goal you listed.

_____

_____

_____

Physical Activity Crossword

Activity B

Chapter 15

Name _____

Date _____ Period _____

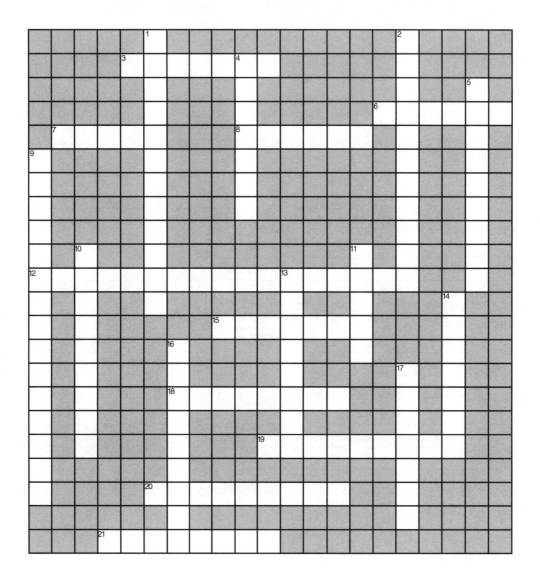

(Continued)

Name_____

Across

3. The position of your body when standing or sitting.
6. *Aerobic* means "with _____."
7. The quickness with which you are able to complete a motion.
8. This heart rate zone is the range of heartbeats at which the heart muscle receives its best workout.
12. The body's _____ fitness describes its ability to take in oxygen and carry it through the blood to body cells.
15. Your ability to keep your body in an upright position.
18. How long an exercise session lasts.
19. How hard you exercise.
20. Activities in which your muscles need more oxygen than your heart and lungs can provide.
21. The ability of the muscles to move objects.

Down

1. The ability to integrate the use of two or more parts of the body.
2. The ability to move your joints through a full range of motion.
4. Your _____ heart rate is the speed at which your heart muscle contracts when you are sitting quietly.
5. Another name for pulse rate.
9. A state in which all body systems function together efficiently.
10. How often you exercise.
11. The ability to do maximum work in a short time.
13. Your _____ time is the amount of time it takes you to respond to a signal.
14. The ability to change body position with speed and control.
16. The ability to use a muscle group over and over without becoming tired.
17. Your _____ heart rate is the highest heart rate at which the heart muscle is able to contract.

The Physical Activity Runaround

Activity C   Name _____

Chapter 15   Date_____ Period _____

Review chapter concepts as you play the game below. Use buttons for markers. Flip a coin to move around the board—"heads" move two spaces; "tails" move one. When you land on a "Turning Point," flip the coin twice on your next turn. The first flip will determine which direction you will go. The second flip will determine how many spaces you will move. Keep a running total of your points on the Fitness Quotient (FQ) Board. The winner is the person with the most points when someone reaches "Finish."

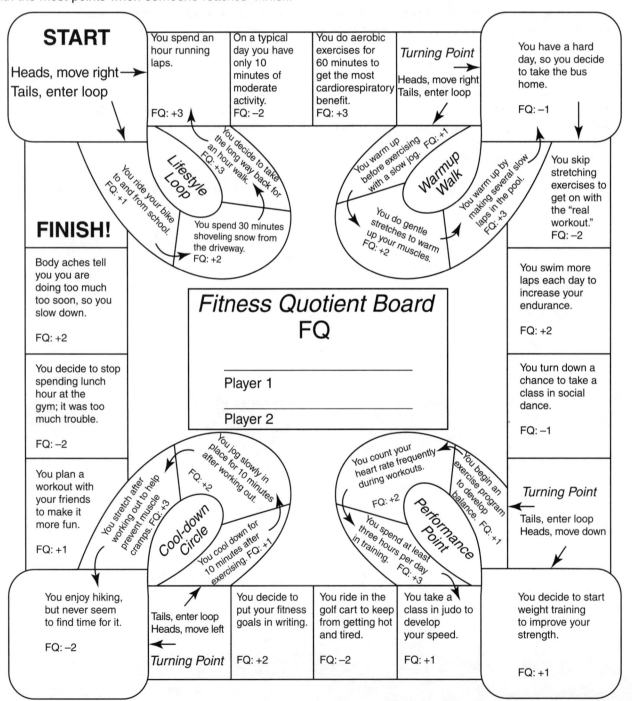

Backtrack
Through Chapter 15

Activity D

Chapter 15

Name _____

Date_____ Period _____

Provide complete answers to the following questions and statements about physical activity.

Recall the Facts
- -

1. List the three main goals for physical activity. _____

    _____

2. How much moderate activity is required per day to achieve good health?_____

3. How can exercise improve posture? _____

    _____

4. Exercise can lower the risk of developing some diseases. Name four. _____

    _____

5. List the five components of physical fitness._____

    _____

6. Give three examples of aerobic activity. _____

7. Give three examples of anaerobic activity. _____

8. List three activities that can build muscle endurance._____

    _____

9. What is body composition? _____

    _____

10. Give an example to demonstrate how speed can help in daily living. _____

    _____

    _____

11. Name four keys to a successful exercise program._____

    _____

12. Name two signs you are working out too hard._____

13. What are the three phases of a workout session? _____

    _____

Interpret Implications
- -

14. Why should people of all body types and sizes consider the benefits of physical activity for weight management?

    _____

(Continued)

Name_____

15. Explain why anaerobic activities do not increase cardiorespiratory fitness._____

_____

_____

16. Why does a slower heartbeat indicate increased fitness?_____

_____

_____

17. How does exercise affect cholesterol levels?_____

_____

Apply & Practice

18. Write one fitness goal for yourself. Then list the steps you could take to achieve this goal.

_____

_____

_____

_____

_____

_____

_____

19. Make a list of physical activities you enjoy. Then make a second list of physical activities you have never tried. Place a check by those you *think* you might enjoy._____

_____

_____

_____

_____

_____

_____

_____

20. Calculate your maximum heart rate and your target heart rate zone. Show your work._____

_____

_____

_____

_____

_____

Eating for Sports Performance

40-Fact Relay

Activity A

Chapter 16

Name _____

Date_____ Period _____

See if you can recognize facts from falsehoods in this challenging "40-Fact Relay." If the statement is true, write the word "True" in the blank. If the statement is false, change the underlined word(s) to make the statement true. Write the corrected word(s) in the blank.

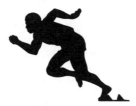

_____ 1. Sports activities help people grow socially and <u>emotionally</u>.

_____ 2. Most low-weight athletes tend to burn <u>more</u> calories through a given type of exercise activity than athletes who weigh more.

_____ 3. More vigorous activities require <u>more</u> energy than less active sports.

_____ 4. Weight is lost whenever an athlete consumes <u>more</u> calories than he or she burns.

_____ 5. Athletes need to take in <u>more</u> calories than nonathletes to maintain their body size.

_____ 6. Athletes need <u>only a small</u> selection of nutritious foods.

_____ 7. Fat <u>is not</u> burned for energy during aerobic activity.

_____ 8. <u>Glucose</u> is the body's chief source of energy.

_____ 9. The body breaks down simple sugar into <u>oxygen</u>, water, and energy.

_____ 10. Lactic acid builds up in the muscles from lack of <u>oxygen</u> to break down glucose.

_____ 11. Athletes <u>can</u> train their muscles to improve the use of glucose.

_____ 12. Endurance athletes learn to pace themselves to maintain the flow of oxygen for steady <u>glucose</u> metabolism.

_____ 13. Athletes need a diet that is high in <u>protein</u> and low in fat.

_____ 14. Athletes <u>need</u> vitamin supplements in order to convert carbohydrates, fats, and proteins to energy.

(Continued)

Name_____

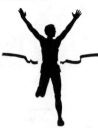

_____15. Dried fruits and yogurt shakes <u>are</u> good concentrated sources of energy for athletes.

_____16. Carbohydrate loading means eating a <u>high-protein</u> diet for several days followed by a high-carbohydrate diet.

_____17. Rest days <u>can</u> help athletes build up glycogen stores.

_____18. The most critical nutritional need of athletes is <u>fluid</u> intake.

_____19. Most performing athletes feel <u>more</u> thirsty during a workout.

_____20. Athletes can see how much water they lose by <u>weighing</u> before and after events.

_____21. It is common for athletes to lose <u>four to six pounds</u> of water weight during an event.

_____22. High humidity tends to <u>increase</u> the amount of water lost during exercise.

_____23. <u>Fruit juice</u> is the preferred liquid for fluid replacement during athletic events.

_____24. Some sports drinks cause cramping because of the <u>carbohydrates</u> they contain.

_____25. Caffeine and alcohol tend to <u>decrease</u> body water loss.

_____26. Using salt tablets is a <u>good</u> way to replenish sodium lost by sweating.

_____27. Pregame meals should provide <u>large</u> amounts of food.

_____28. A good pregame meal should be high in <u>protein</u> and low in fat.

_____29. When an athlete is <u>overweight</u>, energy for competition is used to keep warm.

_____30. The acceptable level of body fat for female athletes is <u>greater</u> than for male athletes.

_____31. Weight lifters <u>strengthen</u> their endurance by avoiding fluids two days before an event.

_____32. Standard practice for training wrestlers <u>does</u> involve the use of laxatives and emetics to reduce body weight prior to competition.

_____33. The best time for athletes to diet is just before <u>competition</u> begins.

_____34. <u>Rapid</u> weight loss is the best way to lose unwanted pounds.

_____35. Consuming 3,500 fewer calories than are expended results in the loss of <u>one pound</u>.

_____36. Athletes who need to gain weight should increase intake by 2,500 calories per <u>day</u>.

_____37. For underweight athletes, weight gain without exercise results in <u>muscle</u> gain.

_____38. Athletes who need to gain or lose weight should work with a registered <u>dietitian</u>.

_____39. Athletes <u>can</u> trust the claims of many sports performance enhancers.

_____40. A planned program of supervised training and nutrition is the <u>safest, most effective</u> key to peak athletic performance.

Analyze This

Activity B   Name _____

Chapter 16   Date_____ Period _____

Read a news or feature article from a current general or fitness-related magazine that deals with eating for sports performance. Then, complete the following analysis of the article based on what you have learned from this chapter.

1. Title of the article: _____

2. Author(s) of the article: _____

3. Title and date of the publication: _____

4. Page numbers: _____

5. What is the focus of the article? _____

   _____

   _____

6. Is the article well written? Why or why not? _____

   _____

   _____

   _____

   _____

7. Give two examples of how studying the chapter helped you understand the subject presented in the article.

   _____

   _____

   _____

   _____

8. Give two examples of new information or ideas you gathered from the article. _____

   _____

   _____

9. Based on your study of the chapter, did the article seem to be misleading or inaccurate? Explain. _____

   _____

   _____

   _____

   _____

10. Would you recommend this article to a friend? Why or why not?_____

   _____

   _____

Ask an Athlete

Activity C

Name _____

Chapter 16

Date _____ **Period** _____

Use the questions below as a guide for interviewing an athlete of your choice. Record the athlete's responses, but not his or her name. Be prepared to discuss the benefits and/or dangers of the performance practices you find.

1. What type of sports do you perform? _____

2. What foods do you eat or avoid just before an event? Why? _____
   _____

3. What steps do you take to increase your endurance? _____
   _____

4. What foods do you eat for energy? _____
   _____

5. What do you prefer to drink before, during, and after a sporting event? _____
   _____

6. Have you ever tried to gain or lose weight to improve your athletic performance? If so, what changes did you make? _____
   _____
   _____
   _____

7. Have you ever taken any type of pill or drink to try to enhance athletic performance? If so, what were the results? _____
   _____
   _____
   _____

Based on your interview, would you classify this athlete as very conscious, somewhat conscious, or not very conscious of eating for sports performance? Explain._____
_____
_____
_____

Based on what you have learned, suggest two ways the athlete you interviewed could improve his or her habits regarding eating for sports performance._____
_____
_____
_____

Backtrack
Through Chapter 16

Activity D

Chapter 16

Name _____

Date _____ Period _____

Provide complete answers to the following questions and statements about eating for sports performance.

Recall the Facts

1. Name five purposes of sports. _____
   _____
   _____

2. What has increased the spread of nutrition myths and misinformation among athletes? _____
   _____

3. What does the body need to enable it to convert glucose into carbon dioxide, water, and energy? _____
   _____
   _____

4. Why are fats considered an almost unlimited source of energy? _____
   _____

5. What is lactic acid and how does it affect the body? _____
   _____

6. Why do athletes need to eat foods that are rich in vitamins and minerals? _____
   _____

7. What problems can occur when athletes practice carbohydrate loading? _____
   _____

8. What are the symptoms of dehydration? _____
   _____

9. How much water is generally lost per hour by sweating during a vigorous workout? _____

10. What fluid intake is recommended by the American Dietetics Association before, during, and after an athletic event? _____
    _____
    _____
    _____

11. What are some reasons why salt tablets are not recommended to replace sodium lost during physical activity? _____
    _____

(Continued)

Name_____

12. How many hours before a game should a pregame meal be eaten?_____

13. What can you conclude about claims of performance enhancers that sound too good to be true? _____

_____

Interpret Implications

14. Explain why the calorie needs of athletes are greater than those of nonathletes. _____

_____

_____

15. Explain what it means when an athlete "hits the wall." _____

_____

_____

16. Explain how percentage of body fat affects athletic performance. _____

_____

17. List one type of performance aid sometimes used by athletes. Explain why this performance aid can have harmful effects and suggest a healthful alternative. _____

_____

_____

_____

18. Explain why an athlete might be concerned with gaining or losing weight. What additional considerations do athletes have when trying to lose, gain, or maintain body weight? _____

_____

_____

Apply & Practice

19. Plan a menu for a pre-event lunch for a weight lifter. _____

_____

_____

_____

_____

20. Plan a menu for a pregame breakfast for a hockey player._____

_____

_____

_____

_____

Maintaining Positive Social and Mental Health

Applying Maslow's Hierarchy

Activity A

Chapter 17

Name _____

Date _____ Period _____

On the pyramid diagram, write the name for each level of Maslow's hierarchy of human needs. Then write in two examples for each type of need. Finally, answer the questions on the next page.

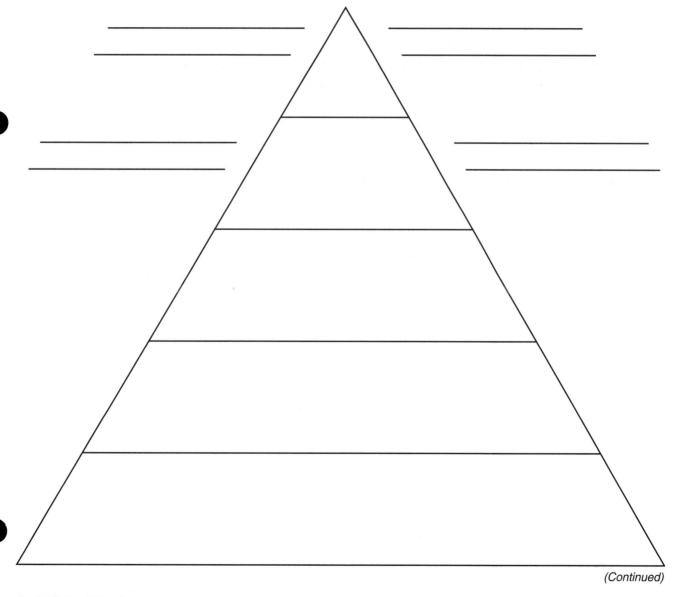

(Continued)

Name_____

1. Why is addressing self-actualization needs important? _____

_____

_____

_____

2. If a person's love and acceptance needs are unmet in childhood, how can this affect the person? What can he or she do to fill these unmet needs? _____

_____

_____

_____

3. Explain how safety and security needs can be threatened by living in a dangerous neighborhood. How can a person feel more safe in this type of environment? _____

_____

_____

_____

4. If a person cannot address physical needs, how does this affect the person's ability to meet self-actualization needs?_____

_____

_____

_____

5. Explain how people can satisfy their esteem needs. _____

_____

_____

_____

Communication Snapshot

Activity B   Name _____

Chapter 17   Date_____ Period _____

Given below are parts of a conversation between a group of students. For each person's communication, circle whether it was ineffective or effective and explain why. Then suggest what the person could have done differently to improve communication.

1. Brian knew his debate teammates wouldn't like what he had to say. He'd thought about what to say and said it just like he planned. "I know our competition is next week, and you have all been counting on me to be there. We've had two resignations at Dad's store, so now I have to work that day. I'm really sorry."

   Ineffective   Effective

   Rationale: _____

   _____

   Suggestion: _____

   _____

2. Without pausing to think, Gerald blurted out, "Deserter!" After that, he refused to speak to Brian any more that day.

   Ineffective   Effective

   Rationale: _____

   _____

   Suggestion: _____

   _____

3. Looking down at her notebook, Susan moaned, "What a mess!"

   Ineffective   Effective

   Rationale: _____

   _____

   Suggestion: _____

   _____

4. Samantha asked, "Are you saying you've made every effort possible to find someone to work in your place?"

   Ineffective   Effective

   Rationale: _____

   _____

   Suggestion: _____

   _____

(Continued)

Name_____

5. Rolling his eyes toward the ceiling, Josh said, "It must have been a tough choice for you."

   Ineffective   Effective

   Rationale: _____

   _____

   Suggestion: _____

   _____

6. Tamika mumbled, "Whatever..."

   Ineffective   Effective

   Rationale: _____

   _____

   Suggestion: _____

   _____

7. Jeremy said, "I've listened to what you said. I'm disappointed, but I understand your dilemma. You must be feeling really bad."

   Ineffective   Effective

   Rationale: _____

   _____

   Suggestion: _____

   _____

8. With a sad look on her face, Patricia said, "Do you think we care if you mess this up for us? We didn't want you to go anyway."

   Ineffective   Effective

   Rationale: _____

   _____

   Suggestion: _____

   _____

Dear Peacemaker

Activity C

Chapter 17

Name _____

Date_____ Period _____

Pretend you write a column called "Dear Peacemaker" for a local newspaper. The column gives readers advice about positive conflict resolution skills. Use the space provided to answer the following letters from your readers about their conflict concerns.

Dear Peacemaker,

I am disgusted with my friend for being so selfish. Whenever we hang out together, we always have to do what he wants and go where he wants—you get the picture. For once, I wish we could do something I like! But I'm afraid to say anything. I don't want to make him mad or hurt his feelings.

"Doormat in Decatur"

Dear Doormat,

_____
_____
_____
_____
_____
_____

Peacemaker

Dear Peacemaker,

I have a big problem with my mom. She always treats me like I am still a three-year-old. When I try to tell her about it, she gets very upset and gives me all kinds of grief. She brings up all the times I was late coming in, got a ticket for speeding, didn't clean my room—you name it! All I want is to be treated like the young adult I am!

"Feeling Grown in Grovetown"

Dear Grown,

_____
_____
_____
_____
_____
_____

Peacemaker

Dear Peacemaker,

I thought brothers were supposed to be close. I can't wait till my brother leaves home for college. He stays on my case about everything—like borrowing his new cap without asking and playing my music too loud when he's studying! He is so unreasonable. No one could please a brother who is that picky! Why do I even bother? I have my own life to live.

"No Bother Brother"

Dear Brother,

_____
_____
_____
_____
_____

Peacemaker

Dear Peacemaker,

My friend and I are not getting along very well lately. She made me really mad, but I didn't tell her. I just got madder and madder on the inside. Then, one day, I blew up at her and said lots of things I really didn't mean. Now she doesn't want to be my friend anymore. Is there anything I can do to make this situation better?

Snapdragon

Dear Snapdragon,

_____
_____
_____
_____
_____

Peacemaker

Teams Work

Activity D   **Name** _____

Chapter 17   **Date**_____ **Period** _____

Take a closer look at the advantages of teamwork by examining the TEAM acronym— "Together Everyone Accomplishes More!" Answer the questions related to each word in the acronym in the spaces provided.

Together

1. What does it mean to cooperate? _____
   _____

2. What does it mean to compromise? _____
   _____

3. Specifically, how can members of a team encourage one another? _____
   _____

Everyone

4. Why is each person's job important to the success of the team?_____
   _____

5. How can members respond if one team member is not doing his or her share?_____
   _____

6. How can members treat others as valued members of the team?_____
   _____

Accomplishes

7. How should groups establish common goals? _____
   _____

8. How can groups be assured team goals will be reached? _____
   _____

More!

9. Why are teams often more effective than individuals? _____
   _____

10. Why are complex problems best addressed by groups? _____
    _____

Countdown to Mental Health

Activity E   **Name** _____

Chapter 17   **Date** _____ **Period** _____

Read each question below and check the appropriate column. Then answer the questions at the bottom of the page.

	Usually	Sometimes	Never
Do you...			
1. surround yourself with people who are supportive?			
2. find role models to serve as good examples?			
3. connect with encouraging friends?			
4. avoid negative thoughts about yourself?			
5. protect your physical health?			
6. eat nutritious foods?			
7. get plenty of rest?			
8. get regular physical activity?			
9. avoid harmful substances?			
10. devote enough time and energy to each of your roles?			

11. For how many responses did you check the "Usually" column? _____

12. For how many responses did you check the "Never" column? _____

13. What do you think this indicates about your mental health?_____

    _____

14. Select one item you think you could improve. Write the number here._____

15. List three goals you could set to address this area. _____

    _____

    _____

    _____

Managing Myself

Activity F   **Name** _____

Chapter 17   **Date**_____ **Period** _____

Prepare a self-management plan for making a positive behavior change in your life. Follow the steps outlined below and fill in the chart.

List your strengths _____   _____ _____   _____
List your improvements needed in order of importance (   )_____   (   )_____ (   )_____   (   )_____
Clarify your goal Express your most-needed improvement as a specific goal. _____ _____
List the alternatives for achieving your goal Indicate advantages and disadvantages of each option. _____ _____ _____ _____ _____
Make a choice and act on it Choose the alternative that seems best. Write it below. Act on it. _____ _____
Evaluate outcomes Analyze the results of your actions. _____ _____ _____

Backtrack
Through Chapter 17

Activity G

Chapter 17

Name _____

Date_____ Period _____

Provide complete answers to the following questions and statements about social and mental health.

Recall the Facts

1. What is a hierarchy? _____

2. Where do the closest and most lasting social relationships occur for most people? _____

3. What other group of people in your social circle serves as a valuable source of self-discovery? _____

4. What type of communication involves the use of spoken or written words?_____

5. What type of communication sends messages without using words? _____

6. For the following "you" message, give a corresponding "I" message: "You make me so mad when you say you will call but don't." _____

_____

7. What is assertiveness? _____

_____

8. Name five characteristics of effective teams. _____

_____

_____

9. What is your personality? _____

_____

10. What five main types of roles do most people have? _____

_____

11. List three questions that can help you evaluate the outcomes of a self-management plan. _____

_____

_____

_____

12. What does burnout mean? _____

_____

13. When social and mental health problems are too great to be solved with self-help techniques, what should a person do? _____

(Continued)

Name_____

Interpret Implications

14. Explain Maslow's rationale for the theory that lower-level needs must be met before a person can address higher-level needs. Give an example to support your explanation._____

_____

_____

_____

15. Explain the link between self-awareness and social health._____

_____

16. Explain the influential role a caregiver can have in a child's social development. What implications does this have for parents who are selecting a child care arrangement for their children? _____

_____

_____

17. Explain the difference between assertive and aggressive. _____

_____

_____

18. Explain the difference between self-concept and self-esteem._____

_____

_____

Apply & Practice

19. Describe in detail someone you know who has positive social and mental health. _____

_____

_____

_____

_____

20. Recall interactions you have observed between people today. List four actions you saw that built self-esteem and four actions you saw that diminished it. _____

_____

_____

_____

_____

_____

_____

_____

Stress and Wellness

18

Do Not Stress Out!

Activity A

Chapter 18

Name _____

Date_____ Period _____

Complete the puzzle by filling in the appropriate terms in the statements below.

1. Minor daily stresses that produce tension are called _____ _____.
2. Someone with a type A _____ tends to be driven to achieve goals.
3. Divorce is an example of a _____-_____ _____, or a major stressor that can greatly alter a person's lifestyle.
4. A technique of focusing on involuntary bodily processes in order to control them is called _____.
5. A reaction in which your body is gathering its resources to conquer danger is a _____ response.
6. The inner agitation you feel when you are exposed to change is _____.
7. A reaction in which your body is gathering its resources to escape to safety is a _____ response.
8. _____ muscle relaxation is a relaxation technique that involves slowly tensing and then relaxing different groups of muscles.
9. Harmful stress is called _____ _____ or distress.
10. A person's internal conversations about himself or herself and the situations he or she faces are called _____-_____.
11. A source of stress is a _____.
12. Stress that motivates you to accomplish challenging goals is _____ _____.
13. A group of people who can provide a person with physical help and emotional comfort is the person's _____ _____.
14. Another name for negative stress is _____.

Copyright Goodheart-Willcox Co., Inc.

127

Stress Metaphors

Activity B   Name _____

Chapter 18   Date_____ Period _____

Consider the following metaphor about stress:

*Stress is like a rubber band...when life
pulls at you, you stretch and give, and
stretch and give, and hope that you don't
POP!*

Use the space below to write your own original metaphor for stress.

Good Stress/Bad Stress

Activity C   **Name** _____

Chapter 18   **Date**_____ **Period** _____

Read the situations below and identify each type of stress as either positive or negative. For each situation of positive stress, identify one good result that could occur. For each situation of negative stress, identify one bad result that could occur.

1. The air was charged with the excitement and anticipation of the crowd. The team ran onto the field for the big game. The crowd cheered, and Jeff, the quarterback, felt a quiver of nervousness race up his spine.

   Type of Stress:_____

   Result: _____

   _____

2. Kara had studied thoroughly for the midterm. As the teacher began to hand out the tests, Kara felt a momentary sense of uncertainty. She took a deep breath and told herself, "Relax, you know this. Just be cool."

   Type of Stress:_____

   Result: _____

   _____

3. Andrew's father is an alcoholic. Andrew never knows when his dad will lose his temper. His dad is more angry these days, and his drinking causes him to miss work. Andrew dreads going home, not knowing what he will find.

   Type of Stress:_____

   Result: _____

   _____

4. Rebecca keeps hearing rumors of impending layoffs at work. Not knowing whether she will lose her job is beginning to wear on her nerves. Rebecca feels anxious and edgy.

   Type of Stress:_____

   Result: _____

   _____

5. Justice is worried. Lately he has noticed physical symptoms that may indicate a serious health problem. The problem runs in his family. He's afraid to go to the doctor, wondering if his worst fears will be realized.

   Type of Stress:_____

   Result: _____

   _____

6. Kendra feels she's between a rock and a hard place. Her dream is to major in veterinary medicine. She also has the chance to receive a full scholarship. To get the scholarship, she must major in pediatric medicine.

   Type of Stress:_____

   Result: _____

   _____

The Pileup Effect

Activity D   **Name** _____

Chapter 18   **Date**_____ **Period** _____

The diagram below illustrates how one stressor leads to a series of other stressors, creating a pileup effect. Once the stress builds so high, it becomes overwhelming. Look at the completed diagram and answer the questions.

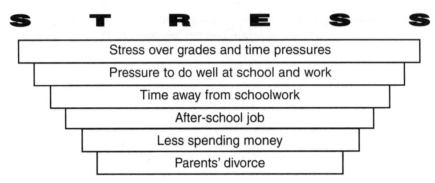

1. What was the core cause of the stress pileup? _____

2. Explain in your own words how the core cause might have caused poor grades as a result of the pileup effect.

   _____

   _____

Now create your own diagram of the pileup effect. At the base of the pyramid, write an example of a core stressor. You may use either a real or imaginary example. At each level, write an example that illustrates how stressors can pile upon one another.

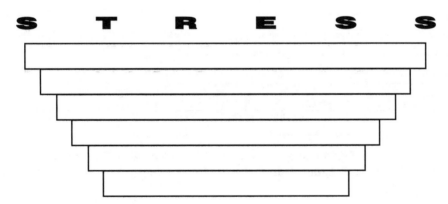

3. List three examples of what a person at the bottom level of the pyramid could have done to alleviate stress.

   _____

   _____

4. How can a person's support system help in alleviating the pileup effect?

   _____

5. Why is it important to deal with smaller stressors before stress has a chance to pile up?

   _____

Straight Talk on Stress

Activity E   Name _____

Chapter 18   Date_____ Period _____

If the statement is true, write the word *true* in the blank. If the statement is false, change the underlined word(s) to make the statement true. Write the correct word(s) in the blank.

_____ 1. The body goes through three stages when it responds to stress—alarm, <u>fight</u>, and exhaustion.

_____ 2. The alarm stage contains both emotional and <u>mental</u> responses.

_____ 3. During the alarm stage, a person's heart rate and blood pressure are likely to <u>increase</u>.

_____ 4. <u>Narrowing</u> of eyes and tensing of muscles are signs the body is preparing either to conquer danger or escape.

_____ 5. During the <u>alarm</u> stage, the stress level starts to subside and muscles begin to relax.

_____ 6. During the <u>exhaustion</u> stage, you may feel tired and unable to concentrate.

_____ 7. Prolonged tension in one area of your life <u>can</u> spill over into other areas.

_____ 8. Chronic stress <u>can</u> lead to physical illness.

_____ 9. Stress can cause physical reactions as stress hormones are released into your <u>brain</u>.

_____ 10. Physical reactions to stress include rapid heartbeat, <u>retention</u> of glucose by the liver, and release of fat cells into the bloodstream.

_____ 11. Increases in heart rate and blood pressure <u>can</u> strain your heart.

_____ 12. Extra fat released into the bloodstream <u>can</u> build up in your arteries.

_____ 13. The immune system's defenses become <u>higher</u> during periods of stress.

_____ 14. During times of stress, your increased level of mental activity can keep you from <u>falling asleep</u>.

_____ 15. When stress hormones are active, your body treats digestion as a <u>high</u> priority.

_____ 16. Stress <u>can</u> be a factor in weight problems and eating disorders.

_____ 17. Your reactions to stress <u>can</u> compromise your nutritional health and, in turn, produce outcomes that compound your stress.

_____ 18. <u>Physical</u> effects of stress include irritability and worry.

_____ 19. Factors that determine how you respond to stressors include <u>heredity</u>, experience, and outlook.

_____ 20. Someone with a type A personality is often more <u>relaxed about</u> stressful events than someone with a type B personality.

Friends in Need

Activity F   **Name** _____

Chapter 18   **Date** _____ **Period** _____

For each scenario below, provide advice to the person under stress. Suggest one positive way the person can manage the stress he or she feels.

1. Shannon is usually a very cheerful person. Lately she has been moody. She has been complaining about headaches and lack of energy. For the past few days, Shannon has not wanted to be around her friends.

_____
_____
_____

2. Theo has been under a lot of stress. He found out his mother has cancer. He has not shared his feelings and fears with his friends. He doesn't want to "bring them down." The school counselor asked to meet with Theo, but Theo managed to find a schedule conflict to avoid the meeting. He just doesn't want to talk about the situation.

_____
_____
_____

3. Holden had waited in a long line of cars to enter the parking lot. Just as it was his turn, another driver cut in front of him and entered the lot first. As Holden inched forward toward the entrance to the parking lot, the "Lot Full" sign appeared.

_____
_____
_____

4. Stacey had always had a hard time with math problems. As she sat down to do her homework, she told herself, "I'm no good at this. I always get more problems wrong than right. I don't know why I even try."

_____
_____
_____

5. Jonathan starts working on assignments early. He loses interest, though, and never seems to finish them until the night before they are due. Sometimes he has to stay up all night, but he always gets them done. Jonathan concludes he works better under pressure.

_____
_____
_____

6. Since she heard about her parents' upcoming divorce, Marita has been depressed. She has stopped taking her daily jog and her appetite has suffered. From the circles under her eyes, it appears she hasn't been sleeping either.

_____
_____
_____

Backtrack
Through Chapter 18

Activity G

Chapter 18

Name _____

Date_____ Period _____

Provide complete answers to the following questions and statements about stress and wellness.

Recall the Facts

1. What feeling usually accompanies stress? _____

2. What are the two types of stress?_____

3. How can negative stress reduce your effectiveness? _____
_____

4. How can positive stress produce good results? _____
_____

5. Is feeling lonely a life-change event or a daily hassle? Why?_____
_____

6. Is moving to a new city a life-change event or a daily hassle? Why?_____
_____

7. What is the flight or fight response? _____
_____

8. Give an example to illustrate each stage of the body's response to stress._____
_____
_____

9. List three serious physical health problems that may result from the effects of stress. _____
_____

10. Name three types of effects stress can have on your physical health._____
_____

11. List five techniques that can help you manage stress. _____
_____
_____

12. List five suggestions for preventing stress by addressing its root causes. _____
_____
_____
_____

13. What is biofeedback? _____
_____

(Continued)

Name_____

Interpret Implications

14. Give one example of a physical stressor and one example of an emotional stressor. Offer a suggestion for alleviating each of these stressors. _____

_____

_____

_____

15. Give an example that illustrates how families in crisis may experience large amounts of stress. _____

_____

_____

16. Explain how a person can use biofeedback to manage stress. _____

_____

_____

17. Explain how a person's support system (or lack of support) can affect his or her ability to handle stress effectively.

_____

_____

18. If a person feels stress due to lack of time, would cutting out leisure activities be a good way to manage this stress? Explain. _____

_____

_____

Apply & Practice

19. Select a common stressor in the lives of teens. Write a paragraph describing causes of the stressor and ways teens can prevent or cope with the stress it creates. _____

_____

_____

_____

_____

_____

20. Write a brief paragraph describing the connection between attitude and stress. Give examples you have observed in real-life situations. _____

_____

_____

_____

_____

_____

The Use and Abuse of Drugs

19

What's the Question?

Activity A

Chapter 19

Name _____

Date_____ Period _____

Listed below are the answers to questions about drug use and abuse. Your task is to write suitable questions in the spaces provided.

1. Prescription and over-the-counter

   Question: _____

2. Reaction caused by a drug along with its intended reaction

   Question: _____

3. Chemical, generic, and trade

   Question: _____

4. Powder, liquid, tablet, caplet, and capsule

   Question: _____

5. Mouth, stomach, or small intestine

   Question: _____

6. Tries to convert toxic chemicals to less toxic substances

   Question: _____

7. Acts as a stimulant and a diuretic

   Question: _____

8. Per day, the equivalent found in two cups of coffee

   Question: _____

9. In appetite suppressants and sleeping pills

   Question: _____

10. When a person requires a larger dose to feel the effects of a drug

    Question: _____

11. Tobacco smoke

    Question: _____

12. Vitamin deficiencies, fat buildup in the liver, and stomach problems

    Question: _____

13. Codeine, morphine, opium, and heroin

    Question: _____

14. Images created by the mind that do not really exist

    Question: _____

15. Synthetic form of testosterone

    Question: _____

Drugs Crossword

Activity B

Chapter 19

Name _____

Date _____ Period _____

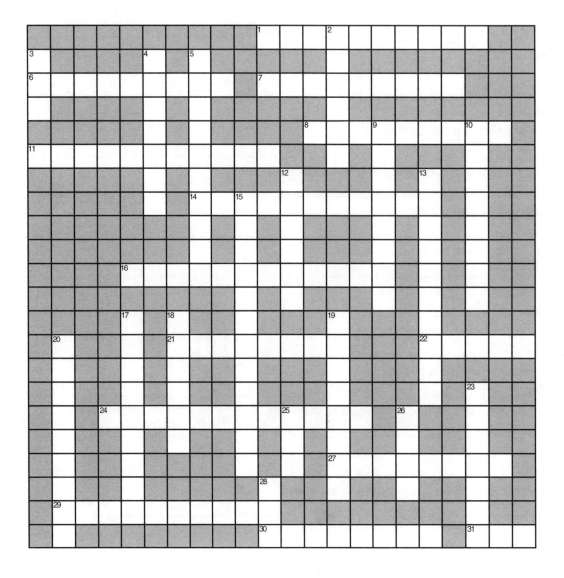

(Continued)

Name_____

Across

1. An addiction to alcohol.
6. A liver disease that often results from alcohol abuse.
7. A psychological or physical dependence on a drug.
8. A psychoactive drug that speeds up the nervous system.
11. A drug without an exclusive brand name.
14. One of several commonly abused stimulant drugs.
16. A drug that causes the mind to create images that do not really exist.
21. A substance that is inhaled for its mind-numbing effects.
22. The use of a drug for a reason other than medical reasons.
24. A drug that can only be obtained from a pharmacy with a written doctor's order.
27. Lab-created imitations of illegal drugs are called _____ drugs.
29. A reaction caused by a drug along with its intended reaction.
30. A mild stimulant drug that is found in coffee, tea, cola, and cocoa products.
31. Abbreviation for lysergic acid diethylamide.

Down

2. A narcotic drug made from the opium poppy.
3. Abbreviation for phencyclidine.
4. A white powdered drug made from the coca plant, usually inhaled through the nose.
5. A set of symptoms experienced by people when they stop taking drugs to which they are addicted.
9. A drug used to treat an ailment or a disabling condition.
10. A drug that brings on sleep, relieves pain, and dulls the senses.
12. Cigarette smoke that is inhaled by people other than the smoker is called _____ hand smoke.
13. A drug that decreases the activity of the central nervous system.
15. Drugs that affect the central nervous system.
17. The ability of the body and mind to refrain from responding to a drug.
18. Use of medicines in ways they were not intended to be used is drug _____.
19. Artificial hormones used to build a more muscular body are anabolic _____.
20. A type of tobacco products that are not intended to be smoked.
23. Drugs that are unlawful to buy or use.
25. The chief mood-altering ingredient in marijuana.
26. The chemical name for the generic drug aspirin is acetylsalicylic _____.
28. Abbreviation for the type of legal drugs that can be obtained without a written doctor's order.

Psychoactive Drugs

Name _____

Date_____ Period _____

Complete the following chart to organize important facts about psychoactive drugs.

Drug	Stimulant, depressant, or hallucinogen?	Sources or uses	Physical effects	Related diseases	Recom-mendations
caffeine					
amphetamines					
cocaine					
nicotine					
alcohol					
barbiturates					
tranquilizers					
inhalants					
narcotics					
marijuana					
LSD/PCP					

Common-Sense Comebacks

Activity D

Chapter 19

Name _____

Date_____ Period _____

Many drug abusers started using and misusing drugs at the urgings of other people. Some people find it hard to turn down an invitation, even when it goes against common knowledge and good sense. Use facts from the chapter to write a good "comeback" or response for each of the invitations below.

1. "How about just one beer to join the party?"

4. "Cigarette smoking isn't addictive. It's just gotten bad press, that's all."

2. "What are you, chicken? It's just glue. One little sniff can't hurt you."

5. "Want to snort some coke with us? It's no big deal. Come on."

3. "You should try these weight control pills. You won't want to eat anything. You'll lose weight and keep it off!"

6. "You need to lighten up. Take just one hit of this pot. It'll make you feel so much better. Just be cool."

What Do You Think?

Activity E   Name _____

Chapter 19   Date_____ Period _____

Respond to the following statements about your opinions on drug use.

Agree   Unsure Disagree

_____ _____ _____ 1. It is wrong to use any illegal drugs.

_____ _____ _____ 2. It's okay to use another person's prescription medicine if he or she gives it to you.

_____ _____ _____ 3. The legal age for buying tobacco products should be lowered.

_____ _____ _____ 4. A person convicted of drinking and driving should have his or her license revoked.

_____ _____ _____ 5. Smoking should be banned in all public places.

_____ _____ _____ 6. It's okay to use illegal drugs if no one finds out about it.

_____ _____ _____ 7. I wish alcohol were illegal for everyone.

_____ _____ _____ 8. Athletes should not be allowed to use anabolic steroids—it gives them an unfair advantage.

_____ _____ _____ 9. All drugs should be legal.

_____ _____ _____ 10. People who sell drugs to children should be put in jail.

_____ _____ _____ 11. The drinking age should be lowered.

_____ _____ _____ 12. People who furnish alcohol or cigarettes to minors should be fined or arrested.

_____ _____ _____ 13. Athletes should be allowed to use anabolic steroids if they want—it's their bodies.

_____ _____ _____ 14. Penalties for driving while drinking should be lowered.

_____ _____ _____ 15. People should stop trying to ban smoking in public.

16. If someone who agreed with statement number _____ wanted to be my friend, I would have to think twice.

    Explain. _____

    _____

    _____

17. If someone I was dating disagreed with statement number _____, I would have to reconsider the relationship.

    Explain. _____

    _____

    _____

18. Final comments on drug use and abuse: _____

    _____

    _____

Backtrack
Through Chapter 19

Activity F

Chapter 19

Name _____

Date_____ Period _____

Provide complete answers to the following questions and statements about drug use and abuse.

Recall the Facts

1. Why are doctors the only people who can write drug prescriptions? _____
_____

2. Is a brand name drug better than the same drug in generic form? Why or why not? _____
_____

3. How do prices of brand name drugs compare with those of generic drugs? _____
_____

4. List five factors that affect the way the body uses the chemicals from drugs. _____
_____

5. What is the difference between drug misuse and drug abuse? _____
_____

6. What are the three main types of psychoactive drugs? _____
_____

7. Name seven symptoms of drug withdrawal. _____
_____

8. Of the drugs described in the chapter, which one kills the most people? _____

9. By how many minutes is a person's life shortened with each cigarette smoked? _____

10. How much extra vitamin C do smokers need, and why? _____
_____

11. If a person is trying to quit smoking, is smokeless tobacco a good substitute? Why or why not? _____
_____

12. Why are designer drugs especially dangerous? _____

13. Name three community resources that can help alcoholics and their families. _____
_____

Interpret Implications

14. What are the symptoms of caffeine withdrawal and how can they be minimized?_____
_____
_____

(Continued)

Name_____

15. Why have amphetamines been found largely ineffective for weight control? _____
_____
_____

16. Explain the effects of tar that collects in the lungs of smokers. _____
_____
_____

17. Explain why many alcoholics find it difficult to get help. _____
_____

18. Explain why the use of anabolic steroids can be dangerous. _____
_____
_____
_____

Apply & Practice

19. List five tips for consumers buying OTC drug products. _____
_____
_____
_____
_____

20. Write a short paragraph describing how you would feel and what you would do if you knew someone close to you was misusing or abusing drugs.
_____
_____
_____
_____
_____

Keeping Food Safe

Safe Shopping List

Activity A

Chapter 20

Name _____

Date _____ Period _____

Read the following food shopping scenarios. Use ideas from the scenarios to help you develop a list of tips for safe food shopping. Record your list of tips in the space provided.

Scenario 1:

A foul odor greeted Jeremy in the produce section at Super Market. He had trouble finding fresh broccoli that looked good. Instead, Jeremy went to the frozen foods case to get frozen broccoli. There he found some broccoli spears, but all the packages were covered with frost! As a last resort, Jeremy decided to serve string beans instead of broccoli and headed for the canned goods aisle.

Scenario 2:

Donnie stopped at Buy Mart to pick up some deli foods for the family picnic. His sister had said the store appeared sloppy, but it was a convenient place to stop on the way to the lake. He noticed some of the cartons of potato salad had expired dates and others had no labels. A few had loosened lids or were stacked well above the level of cold air in the case. Donnie was careful to select only those with current dates and tightly closed lids. He also chose cartons that were stored deep down in the case.

Scenario 3:

Jan heard about the weekend specials at the Corner Grocery. When she reached the back of the store, she started having second thoughts. The meat case was stained with meat drippings. She did not see the cuts she needed in the meat case, but no one was on duty to help her. Finally, she picked a package of cut-up chicken and went to the checkout. Only after she got home did she realize the chicken had leaked all over her lettuce. What a mess!

SAFE SHOPPING

Food at Home and on the Go

Activity B   Name _____

Chapter 20   Date_____ Period _____

Read the following statements about food handling practices at home and away from home. If the statement is true, write the word *true* in the blank. If the statement is false, change the underlined word(s) to make the statement true. Write the correct word(s) in the blank.

_____ 1. Store eggs on the shelf located <u>on the door</u> of the refrigerator.

_____ 2. When you get home from the store, put away <u>perishable</u> foods first.

_____ 3. Keep the refrigerator at a temperature of <u>0</u>°F.

_____ 4. Keep a <u>meat</u> thermometer in your freezer to ensure a safe temperature.

_____ 5. Store dry beans in <u>the refrigerator</u>.

_____ 6. Chill cooked foods <u>quickly</u> to minimize growth of bacteria.

_____ 7. <u>Air circulation</u> helps foods chill more quickly.

_____ 8. Most leftovers will keep safely in the refrigerator for <u>three to four weeks</u>.

_____ 9. <u>Wax paper</u> and plastic wrap are suitable disposable food covers.

_____ 10. The sink base cabinet <u>is</u> a good place to store potatoes and onions.

_____ 11. Wash hands with soap and warm water for <u>20</u> seconds before handling food.

_____ 12. You <u>do</u> need to wash your hands after each time you cough or sneeze.

_____ 13. Wear gloves in the kitchen when you have a <u>cold</u>.

_____ 14. A <u>plastic</u> cutting board is easier to clean than a wooden one.

_____ 15. <u>Bacteria</u> can grow on the blade of a can opener if it is not kept clean.

_____ 16. Dishcloths should be replaced <u>daily</u>.

_____ 17. Bacteria grow <u>least</u> rapidly at temperatures between 60°F and 125°F.

_____ 18. Cooking temperatures <u>will</u> kill most bacteria.

_____ 19. Refrigerate leftovers <u>only after cooling to room temperature.</u>

_____ 20. The safest place to thaw foods is <u>on the kitchen counter</u>.

_____ 21. It is a good idea to <u>taste</u> meat before serving to be sure it is completely done.

_____ 22. Undercooked eggs may contain <u>E. coli</u> bacteria.

_____ 23. Microwave ovens tend to cook foods <u>less</u> evenly than regular ovens.

_____ 24. Pack food to go in an <u>insulated</u> bag or cooler.

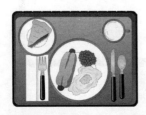

The Contaminators

Activity C

Chapter 20

Name _____

Date_____ Period _____

Choose the best response. Write the letter in the space provided.

_____ 1. Which of the following is true regarding foodborne illness?

A. It is also called food poisoning.
B. It is often mistaken for the "stomach flu."
C. It occurs in millions of people in the United States each year.
D. All of the above.

_____ 2. Single-celled microorganisms that live in soil, water, and the bodies of plants and animals are called _____.

A. protozoa
B. viruses
C. parasites
D. bacteria

_____ 3. A _____ is an organism that lives off a host organism.

A. protozoan
B. virus
C. parasite
D. bacterium

_____ 4. A disease-causing agent that is the smallest type of life-form is a _____.

A. protozoan
B. virus
C. parasite
D. bacterium

_____ 5. *E. coli* is a type of _____.

A. protozoan
B. virus
C. parasite
D. bacterium

_____ 6. *Trichinella* is a type of _____.

A. protozoan
B. virus
C. parasite
D. bacterium

_____ 7. *Hepatitis A* is a type of _____.

A. protozoan
B. virus
C. parasite
D. bacterium

_____ 8. Reactions to illness-causing bacteria _____.

A. vary from one person to another
B. are affected by one's genetic makeup
C. are affected by one's state of health
D. All of the above.

_____ 9. Which of the following is at lowest risk of foodborne illness?

A. Adolescents.
B. Alcoholics.
C. Elderly people.
D. Pregnant females.

_____10. The most common symptoms of foodborne illness are _____.

A. vomiting, skin rash, and headache
B. chills, diarrhea, and headache
C. dizziness, vomiting, and fatigue
D. vomiting, diarrhea, and stomach cramps

(Continued)

Name_____

_____11. Symptoms of most foodborne illness _____.

A. appear within a few hours and last less than one day
B. appear within a day or two and last a few days
C. appear within a week or two and last a few days
D. appear within 30 days and last a few weeks

_____12. When you are in doubt about the safety of a food, _____.

A. take a small bite to see if it has an off taste
B. check to see if it smells spoiled
C. bring it to a boil to kill the bacteria
D. None of these.

_____13. For mild symptoms of foodborne illness, _____.

A. call the doctor immediately
B. drink lots of fluids and rest
C. eat lots of fiber and rest
D. take aspirin and drink lots of fluids

_____14. Symptoms of severe foodborne illness are _____.

A. fever, blood in stools, dehydration, and dizziness
B. cramps, vomiting, diarrhea, and fever
C. dizziness, headache, fever, and chills
D. diarrhea, abdominal pain, and headache

_____15. Double vision, inability to swallow, and difficulty speaking are symptoms of _____.

A. E. coli poisoning
B. toxicity
C. botulism
D. trichinosis

_____16. You should file a report of a foodborne illness if the food _____.

A. came from a public source
B. was served to a large number of people
C. was a commercial product
D. All of the above.

_____17. Which of the following is the correct sequence for the food chain?

A. Food consumers, food producers, food processors, and government agencies.
B. Food processors, food producers, consumers, and government agencies.
C. Food producers, food processors, government agencies, and consumers.
D. Farmers, food consumers, food processors, and government agencies.

_____18. Safe use of pesticides is a responsibility of _____.

A. food processors
B. food producers
C. consumers
D. All of the above.

_____19. The government agency that regulates food advertising is _____.

A. Department of Agriculture
B. Federal Trade Commission
C. Environmental Protection Agency
D. Food and Drug Administration

_____20. The government agency that inspects fish products is the _____.

A. FDA
B. EPA
C. USDA
D. NMFS

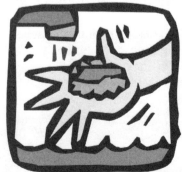

Backtrack
Through Chapter 20

Activity D

Chapter 20

Name _____

Date _____ Period _____

Provide complete answers to the following questions and statements about food safety.

Recall the Facts
- -

1. Why do many cases of foodborne illness go unreported? _____

_____

2. What is the most common cause of foodborne illness in the United States?_____

3. What five types of bacteria cause the most common and/or serious foodborne illnesses?_____

_____

4. What two viruses may be contracted from contaminated raw or undercooked shellfish? _____

_____

5. List five main steps for outwitting food contaminators. _____

_____

_____

6. How can food processors help ensure a safe food supply? _____

_____

_____

7. What foods are monitored by the USDA and FSIS?_____

8. What foods are monitored by the FDA? _____

9. Who checks food handling in local grocery stores and food service operations? _____

_____

10. What are a consumer's responsibilities with regard to food safety?_____

_____

_____

Interpret Implications
- -

11. Can a person avoid foodborne illness completely by avoiding foods that look, smell, and taste bad? Why or why not? _____

_____

12. Is it safe to eat rare pork roast? Why or why not? _____

_____

13. Why should moldy foods be discarded? _____

_____

(Continued)

Name_____

14. If you have many errands, why should you save food shopping for last?_____

_____

15. List two precautions you should take when cooking marinated meats. _____

_____

_____

16. Why are children at greater risk of foodborne illness than adults?_____

_____

17. Why would you want to keep food you suspect has made you ill?_____

_____

Apply & Practice

18. How can you protect yourself from pesticide residues? _____

_____

19. How can you protect yourself from environmental contaminants found in fish?_____

_____

20. What personal hygiene habits have you violated or seen violated by others when working with food?_____

_____

_____

_____

Meal Management

A Meal Manager in the Making

Activity A

Chapter 21

Name _____

Date _____ Period _____

Meg writes in her diary some of her experiences in meal planning and preparation. Identify the advantage of meal planning that is not being realized in each of Meg's entries. Select from the following list: *appeal, nutrition, economy,* and *saving time and effort.* List tips that would have prevented Meg's problems each day and helped her become a better meal manager.

Sept. 2— Our first dinner in the apartment was no picnic! It took all afternoon to cook and most of the evening to clean up the kitchen. I couldn't find anything in that kitchen. I had to stop twice and run down to the convenience store for ingredients I needed. That stuffing recipe had the longest list of ingredients I've ever seen. What are shallots, anyway? I thought the turkey would never get done! I've learned my lesson!

1. Advantage Missing: _____

2. Tips: _____

_____

Sept. 4— Sorry, Diary, but I've been too busy to write. We're having turkey again tonight. Boy, am I tired of turkey sandwiches on white bread. I know we can't afford to waste the turkey, so maybe we can bear it just one more night. I'll boil some potatoes to go with it, and we can have a bowl of vanilla ice cream.

3. Advantage Missing: _____

4. Tips: _____

Sept. 5— Well, it's four for dinner again tonight. Diane won't be here, but Beth is bringing home a friend. The catch is she's a vegetarian—I guess that rules out turkey sandwiches. Maybe I could just fix sandwiches for the rest of us and warm up some canned vegetables for Beth's friend. That sounds like a plan.

5. Advantage Missing: _____

6. Tips: _____

Sept. 6— Since the turkey's finally gone, I stopped by the grocery store today to shop for tonight's dinner. Luckily, I had all the money for this month's food budget with me. I was so hungry! I picked up a few snack items. I couldn't resist the fresh asparagus, even though it was out of season and very expensive. I found four of the best-looking Porterhouse steaks. I thought we could grill outside to keep from heating the apartment. The meal was great. Everyone loved it. The only problem now is how we are going to eat for the rest of the month.

7. Advantage Missing: _____

8. Tips: _____

_____

Meal Makeovers

Activity B

Chapter 21

Name _____

Date_____ Period _____

Each menu below lacks variety in one of the following ways: flavor, color, texture, shape and size, or temperature. For each menu, determine which type of variety is most lacking and write it in the blank under the arrow. Use the block on the right to do a menu makeover that will improve variety.

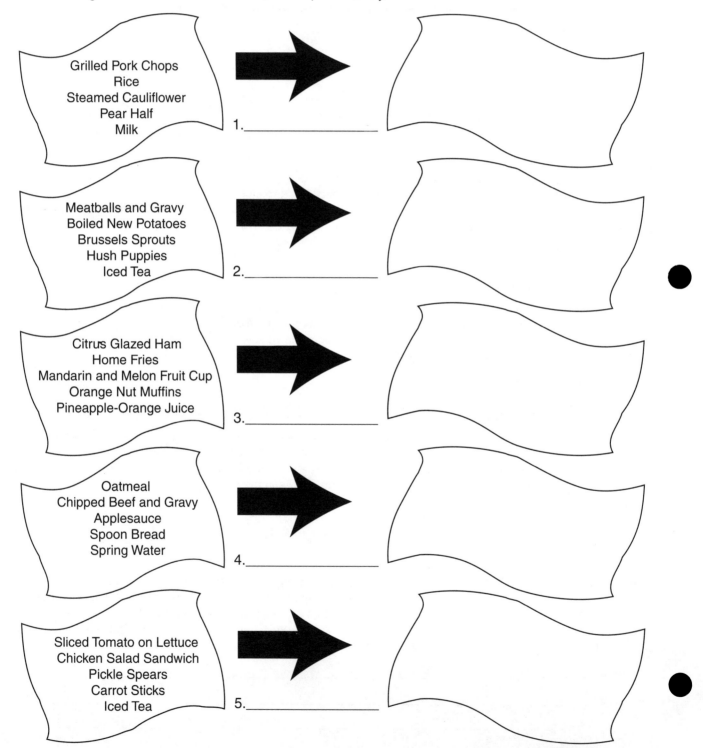

Grilled Pork Chops
Rice
Steamed Cauliflower
Pear Half
Milk

1._____

Meatballs and Gravy
Boiled New Potatoes
Brussels Sprouts
Hush Puppies
Iced Tea

2._____

Citrus Glazed Ham
Home Fries
Mandarin and Melon Fruit Cup
Orange Nut Muffins
Pineapple-Orange Juice

3._____

Oatmeal
Chipped Beef and Gravy
Applesauce
Spoon Bread
Spring Water

4._____

Sliced Tomato on Lettuce
Chicken Salad Sandwich
Pickle Spears
Carrot Sticks
Iced Tea

5._____

Three Squares Plus

Activity C

Chapter 21

Name _____

Date_____ Period _____

A typical way of meeting nutritional needs is to plan three square meals a day plus a nutritious snack. Use the squares provided to plan a nutritious menu for one day using foods you enjoy. Keep in mind lunch and dinner should each supply one-third of your daily nutritional needs. Breakfast should furnish one-fourth of your needs and a snack should provide the rest. Then answer the question at the bottom of the page.

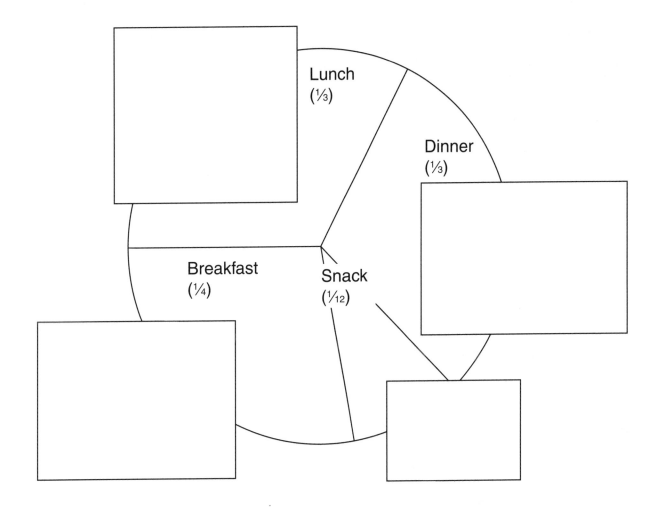

Must everyone follow the "three squares plus" eating pattern each day in order to be healthy? Explain.

_____

_____

_____

Budgeting Dilemmas

Activity D   Name _____

Chapter 21   Date_____ Period _____

Pretend you have budgeted $50 a month for food. This includes eating out and buying any grocery items not purchased by your family. Use your food money wisely. Read each of the following situations and decide what to do. Write your decision about each item before reading any further. Use the notepad on the right to calculate your spending. Then answer the questions about your spending.

1. January 4: A friend invites you to the mall. You are hungry, and Chinese food looks good. The meal you like costs $4.75.

   You decide: _____

2. January 7: You want to start eating yogurt at breakfast. Your family doesn't eat yogurt, so you'll have to buy it. At the grocery store, yogurt costs $3.25 for five containers.

   You decide: _____

3. January 9: At school, you like to buy juice from the vending machine at lunch each day. One carton of juice costs 55 cents. There are 19 school days this month.

   You decide: _____

4. January 11: When your family is visiting a museum, you want lemonade ($2.00) and nachos ($2.50) from the snack bar.

   You decide: _____

5. January 17: You and a date go to a movie. It is your turn to buy refreshments. Your date suggests you each get a medium popcorn and large soft drink. The total price is $9.

   You decide: _____

6. January 18: You're buying snacks for a video party at your house. You can't decide whether to serve a fruit salad or banana splits. In either case, the ingredients cost about $8.

   You decide: _____

7. January 19: You are studying for a test with a friend. Your friend wants to have a pizza delivered. Each of you would pay half (about $7.50).

   You decide: _____

8. January 21: Your mom's birthday is next week. You want to surprise her with a cake. You could make it yourself (ingredients total about $7) or order it specially made from the store bakery ($15).

   You decide: _____

9. January 26: You think about asking a date to dinner. At the restaurant you have chosen, you expect dinner and tip to cost at least $20.

   You decide: _____

10. January 31: On your class field trip, lunch is in the Capitol building restaurant. You can eat: a salad ($2.99); soup and salad, ($3.50); or a hamburger and fries ($4.99).

    You decide: _____

Budget Notebook

January	$50

(Continued)

Name_____

11. At the end of the month, how much had you spent on food? _____

12. How did this compare to the $50 you had budgeted? _____

_____

13. Were there any purchases you made that were poor decisions? Why or why not? _____

_____

_____

14. What other purchases would you have made if you had budgeted more money for food? _____

_____

15. How do the decisions in this activity compare to food decisions you must make in your life? Explain. _____

_____

_____

_____

_____

_____

16. How might setting a food budget help you control your food spending? Explain. _____

_____

_____

_____

_____

Eating Out and About

Activity E

Chapter 21

Name _____

Date _____ Period _____

Eating meals away from home is a challenge for meal managers today. Prepare a list of tips for nutritional eating when you are "out and about" and record tips in the spaces provided. Prepare a menu for a nutritious meal or snack in each category.

Tips for Packing Lunches

Tips for Takeout

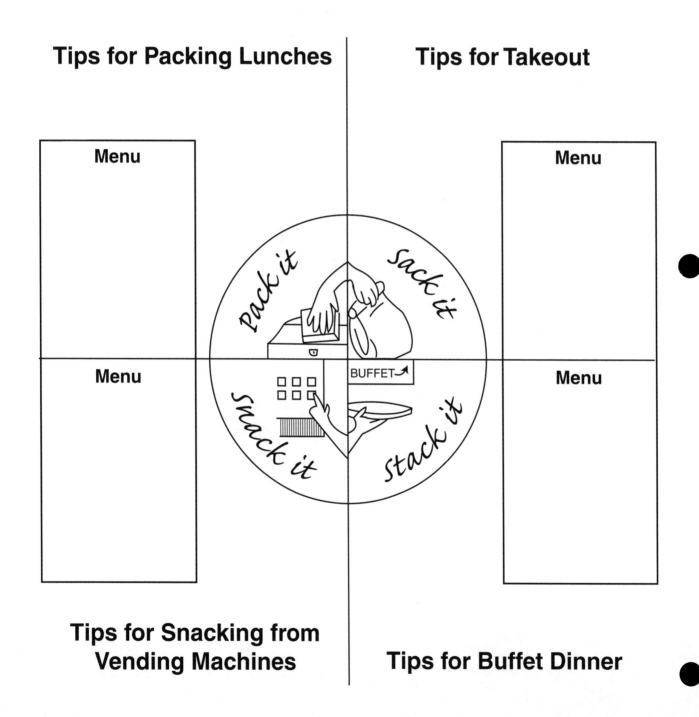

Menu

Menu

Menu

Menu

Tips for Snacking from Vending Machines

Tips for Buffet Dinner

Backtrack
Through Chapter 21

Activity F

Chapter 21

Name _____

Date_____ Period _____

Provide complete answers to the following questions and statements about meal management.

Recall the Facts

1. Name four advantages of planning meals. _____

   _____

2. Name five ways you can add variety to make meals more enjoyable. _____

   _____

3. What resources can meal managers use to help meet nutritional needs?_____

   _____

4. Following the Dietary Guidelines for Americans will help you control what in your diet? _____

   _____

   _____

5. What is a meal pattern? _____

   _____

6. How can using a microwave oven help protect the nutrients in foods? _____

   _____

7. What is a budget? _____

   _____

8. Name five examples of timesaving appliances. _____

   _____

9. What are convenience foods?_____

   _____

10. Name three items you can order in fast-food restaurants to substitute for less-nutritious selections. _____

    _____

Interpret Implications

11. Explain two reasons for serving a variety of foods._____

    _____

(Continued)

Name_____

12. Explain the difference between fixed and flexible expenses and list four examples of each._____

_____

_____

_____

_____

13. List three tips to keep in mind when preparing a food budget._____

_____

_____

14. Name two tools you would store near each of the following locations:

A. sink _____

B. range _____

C. refrigerator _____

D. table _____

15. What are three advantages of convenience foods? _____

_____

16. What are two disadvantages of convenience foods? _____

_____

17. Name an advantage of packed lunches for eating away from home. _____

_____

Apply & Practice

18. List two goals you have related to meal management. List resources that can help you reach each goal.

_____

_____

19. Compare your nutritional needs with those of a family member with different nutritional needs. How does your family manage meals to accommodate these different needs? _____

_____

_____

20. List 10 relatively high-cost foods. For each, list a replacement food from the same food group that is relatively low in cost._____

_____

_____

_____

_____

_____

_____

Making Wise Consumer Choices

22

Where to Shop?

Activity A

Chapter 22

Name _____

Date _____ Period _____

Match the terms with their identifying phrases.

_____ 1. Group of produce stands offered by a group of farmers, often in a city location.

_____ 2. Stores that often sell food items in large containers and multiunit packages.

_____ 3. Grocery stores that may offer many other products and services.

_____ 4. Stores that sell products made by one food manufacturer.

_____ 5. Stores that stay open around the clock so people can stop in quickly and pick up a few items.

_____ 6. Food store that is open only to members who pay an annual fee and volunteer their services.

_____ 7. Produce stand offered by an individual farmer.

A. convenience store

B. cooperative

C. farmers' market

D. outlet store

E. roadside stand

F. specialty store

G. supermarket

H. warehouse store

In the section below, read the shopper's main concern. For each item, write in the type of store the shopper could choose to best satisfy this concern.

_____ 8. Trudy runs every morning before classes. She is interested in a sign she has seen advertising fresh fruits and vegetables for sale in a neighbor's backyard.

_____ 9. Tom is at home late one evening and realizes he is out of bread. He wants to just run in, buy the bread, and get home to make his sandwich.

_____ 10. Amelia wants to shop somewhere that isn't crowded. In fact, she would like a place that is not open to the public.

_____ 11. Carl likes a large selection. He also prefers to have his prescriptions filled while he is shopping.

_____ 12. Armando needs the freshest fruit for a recipe. He lives in the city and doesn't have time to travel far.

_____ 13. Lisa and her husband have seven children. They like to buy frozen foods, peanut butter, and other items in large quantities. This helps them save money.

_____ 14. Keisha prefers to get her meat directly from a butcher because the quality of meat is better.

_____ 15. Kimberly likes to buy a certain brand of bread products. She doesn't mind if the bread is somewhat misshapen—if the price is right.

What Influences Shopping Decisions?

Activity B   Name _____

Chapter 22   Date_____ Period _____

Interview the person in your home who does most of the food shopping for your family. If possible, conduct the interview just after a trip to the store. Record responses below, and share your findings with the class.

Section I.   Advertising as an Influence

1. Think of a specific product you have bought recently. List the item here: _____

    A. Have you seen any advertising on this product? _____

    B. If so, what medium of advertising was used?_____

    C. Do you think the ad had any influence on your decision to buy the product? _____

    D. What type of impression, if any, did the ad make on you?_____

    _____

    E. Did the ad focus on facts about the product? Explain. _____

    _____

    F. Did the ad try to appeal to your basic needs or desires? Did it claim or imply the product could improve your life in some way? Explain. _____

    _____

Section 2.   Form of Food as an Influence

2. Of the following choices, which form of each product do you purchase most often? Circle responses. Explain each choice.

    A. A loaf of bread: Plain white bread   Enriched white bread   Whole-grain bread

    Reason: _____

    B. Green beans: Fresh   Canned   Frozen

    Reason: _____

    C. Chicken: Whole fresh   Cut fresh   Frozen breasts   Cooked, ready-to-eat

    Reason: _____

    D. Butter/margarine: Butter   Regular margarine   Fortified margarine

    Reason: _____

Section 3.   Health as an Influence

3. Do you generally read the ingredient lists and nutritional information on food labels? Why or why not?_____

    _____

4. What food additives, if any, do you try to avoid or minimize in your food purchases? _____

    _____

(Continued)

Name_____

5. Do you buy organic foods? Why or why not? _____

_____

6. Do you wash fruits and vegetables before using? Why or why not?_____

_____

Section 4.   Price as an Influence

7. Do you generally compare prices and quality of similar products before choosing what to buy? Why or why not?

_____

_____

8. Do you use unit pricing information? Why or why not?_____

_____

9. Which do you tend to buy most often—national brands, store brands, or generic products? Explain. _____

_____

10. Do you use a shopping list? _____

A. Is your list organized by category, such as meats, dairy products, and frozen foods? _____

B. Do you plan menus ahead and use these to determine what items to put on the list? _____

C. Do you consult recipes as needed for lists of ingredients to be purchased? _____

D. Do you keep a running list of items needed as you run out of things during the week? _____

E. Do you review advertised specials to aid in making your list? _____

F. Do you often use coupons when shopping for food items? _____

11. Do you tend to purchase items on impulse?_____

A. Do you avoid shopping when you are hungry or tired? _____

B. Do you try to select foods that are in season? _____

C. Do you tend to be drawn to store displays of items not on your shopping list? _____

Design a Label

Name _____

Date_____ Period _____

Imagine you have been hired as a label designer for a well-known distributor of canned foods. Use the sketched outline to create a label that is both visually appealing and in compliance with labeling laws. Think of a creative name for the food distribution company, food product, and brand name. Be sure to include the name and form of the food, the name and address of the distributor, a list of ingredients, and a nutrition panel. Refer to several canned food items for sample label layouts.

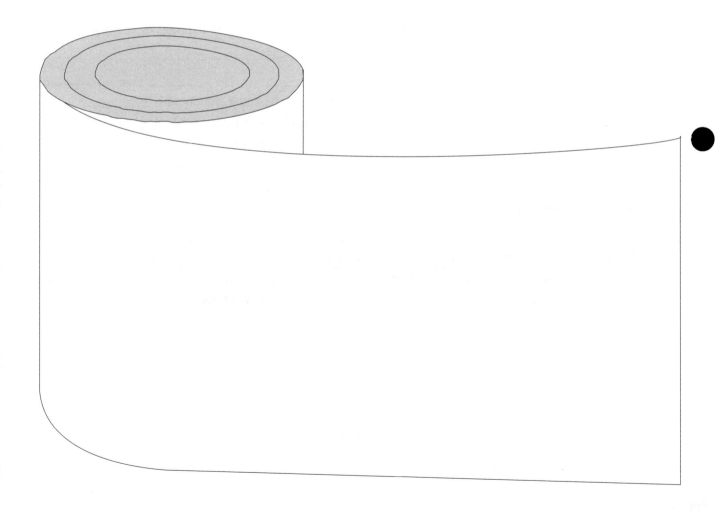

Savvy Shopper or Careless Consumer?

Activity D

Chapter 22

Name _____

Date_____ Period _____

A savvy shopper is knowledgeable about products and uses available information to make informed choices. A careless consumer, on the other hand, does not plan ahead, ask questions, or compare prices and quality. Read the shopping scenarios below. In the blanks on the left, write *SS* each time you read a practice of savvy shopper and *CC* for each illustration of a careless consumer. Use the space beneath each scenario to identify the practice that was either savvy or careless.

_____ 1. Darrin decided to purchase his hiking boots on the Internet. It would be so much easier than fighting crowds at the local mall. He was pretty sure he knew what size to get. He wasn't too concerned by the online store's no refund and no exchange policy.

Practice: _____

_____ 2. Sharonda found a pair of white shorts that fit her perfectly. When she noticed they did not have pockets for her tennis balls, though, she put them back on the rack.

Practice: _____

_____ 3. Abdul told the salesperson he needed new workout clothes that were made of natural fibers that would absorb his body perspiration.

Practice: _____

_____ 4. Kenita usually preferred jogging clothes with a loose fit, but she couldn't resist the bright yellow jogging set. Even though it was a little more snug than she liked, the tag read "Reduced 50%." This was just too good to pass up!

Practice: _____

_____ 5. Donovan was excited when his mom gave him money for his birthday. He decided to buy a new set of golf clubs. The local sporting goods store had sold out of the style he preferred, so he settled for a similar style instead. He did not want to wait for the store to reorder his favorite clubs.

Practice: _____

_____ 6. Gerald decided to spend the $100 he had saved for a home gym. He bought a jump rope, a floor mat, and a variety of hand weights.

Practice: _____

_____ 7. Jan had trouble disciplining herself to work out each day. She decided to invest in a year's membership in a nearby gym. There she could work out six days a week with a class of twelve other people.

Practice: _____

_____ 8. Lorraine considered purchasing an exercise bike to put in her apartment. She read consumer articles about the leading models available and studied features in three nearby stores. Lorraine also talked with several friends who had recently bought exercise bikes.

Practice: _____

_____ 9. Mark hurriedly unpacked his new rowing machine. He threw the instruction booklet aside and started rowing.

Practice: _____

(Continued)

Name_____

_____10. Before he decided which pieces of exercise equipment to buy, Eli measured the space he had. He did a scale drawing of the equipment in his room to check for fit.

Practice:_____

_____11. Maureen saw the weight loss massage belt advertised on television and immediately called the 800 number to order.

Practice:_____

_____12. Jennifer's friends raved about a new workout video. Before deciding whether to order the video, Jennifer went by the library to check out a copy and preview it.

Practice:_____

_____13. Harold's coach advised him to hire a personal trainer to help him prepare for the upcoming weightlifting competition. Harold called the number he saw advertised on the gym bulletin board. He met the trainer, liked him, and hired him on the spot.

Practice:_____

_____14. Cecil found a health club that had just the right set of services to suit his exercise needs. The only problem was the club was 40 minutes from his workplace and 50 minutes from his home. He decided to go ahead and join anyway, thinking somehow he would manage it.

Practice:_____

_____15. Amy did a cost comparison of the YWCA, a nearby spa, and a community fitness center. This helped her select the best facility to meet her needs.

Practice:_____

_____16. John bought a pair of running shoes from a local sports store. Within a week, the inner sole cushions were falling apart. John was very unhappy with the shoes, but he figured that's what happens when you buy inexpensive shoes.

Practice:_____

_____17. Austin attempted to get a refund for a defective air pump he had purchased to inflate a raft. The store refused to refund his money, even though he had his receipt. When Austin contacted the manufacturer, he was told the store should return his money. Austin was unsatisfied, so he contacted a government agency about the problem.

Practice:_____

_____18. Natalie bought a treadmill for running at home. After she got it home, the treadmill did not work properly. Natalie contacted the store where she had made the purchase. Because she had kept her receipt, the store could easily exchange the treadmill.

Practice:_____

_____19. Lucas purchased some boxing gloves for a class he was taking. The week before the first meeting, the class was canceled due to low enrollment. Lucas took his gloves back to the store and demanded a full refund. He did not have a receipt.

Practice:_____

_____20. Monica purchased a month's membership at a gym. When she joined, Monica was unaware the gym's showering facilities were unsafe. Her membership was nonrefundable, so Monica decided there was nothing she could do.

Practice:_____

Backtrack
Through Chapter 22

Activity E

Chapter 22

Name _____

Date _____ Period _____

Provide complete answers to the following questions and statements about food and fitness consumer choices.

Recall the Facts

1. What is a consumer? _____

_____

2. List three advantages food processing offers consumers. _____

_____

_____

3. Give two examples of how food processing can affect the chemical and physical characteristics of food products.

_____

_____

_____

4. Where do manufacturers go to seek approval for the use of food additives?_____

_____

5. Does research support the belief that organic produce is more nutritious than nonorganic? _____

6. Where should you look to find unit price information in the grocery store? _____

_____

7. What two agencies regulate food labeling, and what is the area of responsibility of each? _____

_____

8. What food products are exempt from labeling laws? _____

_____

9. How must ingredients be listed on a label? _____

10. How do consumers use ingredient lists on labels?_____

_____

_____

11. What two items are required for taking part in physical activity? _____

_____

12. What are your rights as a consumer when buying products?_____

_____

(Continued)

Name_____

Interpret Implications

13. Which three of the types of food stores do you think are most popular? For each, give two reasons to support your answer.

_____
_____
_____
_____
_____
_____
_____

14. Give one example explaining why an advertiser might want to use persuasive advertising and one example explaining why an advertiser might want to use informational advertising. _____
_____
_____

15. If organic foods cost so much more than nonorganic foods, why might a person choose to buy them?

_____
_____
_____

16. Explain why the intended use of a food product affects your choice of national brands, store brands, or generic products._____
_____

17. Explain the difference between the *sell by* date and the *use by* date on a food product. _____
_____

18. Name three parties to whom you may need to issue a complaint as a consumer. _____
_____

Apply & Practice

19. Describe how consumers can use the Nutrition Facts panel on a food product label._____
_____
_____

20. Review the shopping pointers for fitness products and services found in this chapter. Select the one that would be the most helpful to you and explain how you could implement it. _____
_____

Food and Fitness Trends

This Word or That

Activity A

Chapter 23

Name _____

Date _____ Period _____

Read each of the following statements. If a statement is true, write *T* in the blank. If a statement is false, select the best word among choices *A* through *D* to substitute for the underlined word to make the statement true. Write the letter of the best choice in the blank.

_____ 1. A <u>change</u> is a general pattern or direction.
  A. norm
  B. trend
  C. plan
  D. form

_____ 2. A <u>trend</u> is a typical pattern.
  A. norm
  B. change
  C. plan
  D. form

_____ 3. The sensation perceived by the tongue during eating is called <u>mouth feel</u>.
  A. olestra
  B. texture
  C. richness
  D. flavor

_____ 4. The first calorie-free fat replacer was <u>chaparral</u>.
  A. Simplesse®
  B. Oatrim
  C. margarine
  D. olestra

_____ 5. <u>Nonnutrient</u> supplements provide no nutritional value, even though they are sold in health food stores.
  A. Protein
  B. Vitamin A
  C. Iron
  D. Vitamin C

_____ 6. A(n) <u>botanical</u> is plant material or part of a plant.
  A. phytochemical
  B. herbal
  C. biological
  D. zoological

_____ 7. A concentrated level of an ingredient many times greater than it occurs naturally in foods is a <u>macrodose</u>.
  A. megadose
  B. maxidose
  C. magnadose
  D. overdose

_____ 8. The science of changing the <u>environmental factors</u> of an organism is called bioengineering.
  A. nutritional content
  B. safety precautions
  C. genetic makeup
  D. historical background

_____ 9. An herbicide is a(n) <u>plant</u> killer used to control weeds.
  A. bacteria
  B. odor
  C. calorie
  D. insect

_____ 10. A weakened strain of a disease-causing organism that is grown in a laboratory is a(n) <u>virus</u>.
  A. culture
  B. vaccine
  C. antibody
  D. phytochemical

(Continued)

Name_____

_____11. The <u>DNA</u> is a government agency in charge of regulating foods and drugs.
  A. RDA
  B. EPA
  C. FDA
  D. FBI

_____12. A high resistance to a disease is called a(n) <u>immunity</u>.
  A. allergy
  B. reaction
  C. inoculation
  D. control

_____13. <u>Useful</u> foods are foods that provide health benefits beyond basic nutrition.
  A. Good
  B. Tasty
  C. Functional
  D. Healthful

_____14. Competitive bacteria prevent the growth of pathogens that cause <u>cancer</u>.
  A. foodborne illness
  B. obesity
  C. eating disorders
  D. allergies

_____15. <u>DNA fingerprinting</u> is used to trace causes of food poisoning.
  A. competitive bacteria
  B. active packaging
  C. irradiation
  D. bioengineering

_____16. <u>Inactive</u> packaging interacts with the food or the atmosphere it contains.
  A. Interactive
  B. Passive
  C. Active
  D. Adaptive

_____17. The return to the manufacturer of defective products is called a <u>recycle</u>.
  A. complaint
  B. precaution
  C. safeguard
  D. recall

_____18. <u>Irradiation</u> is the exposure of food to ionizing energy.
  A. Radiation
  B. Radiology
  C. Photosynthesis
  D. Oxidation

_____19. The <u>service</u> sector employs people who provide assistance.
  A. business
  B. product
  C. volunteer
  D. automation

_____20. People who do a lot of sitting are said to be <u>senile</u>.
  A. obese
  B. sedentary
  C. lazy
  D. hyperactive

Write a short paragraph about food and fitness trends, using seven of the vocabulary words from the chapter.

_____
_____
_____
_____
_____
_____
_____
_____
_____

Assemble the Evidence

Activity B

Chapter 23

Name _____

Date_____ Period _____

In the space provided, give evidence to support each type of trend listed below. Use the text, newspapers, phone directories, the Internet, and other resources as needed.

Trend #1
International Foods and Flavors
- Ethnic Restaurants

_____

_____

_____

- Food Festivals

_____

_____

_____

- TV Cooking Shows

_____

_____

_____

_____

Trend #2
Freshness and Convenience
- New Types of Ready-to-Eat Foods

_____

_____

_____

- Ready-to-Use Fresh Vegetables

_____

_____

_____

- Single-Serving Meals

_____

_____

_____

_____

Trend #3
Lowfat Foods
- Foods with Fat Replacers

_____

_____

_____

_____

Trend #4
Nonnutrient Supplements
- Products with No Nutritional Value Claiming to Promote Health

_____

_____

_____

_____

Comparing Nonnutrient Supplements

Activity C   Name _____

Chapter 23   Date_____ Period _____

Go to a local store that sells nonnutrient supplements. Compare two brands of the same nonnutrient supplement. For each item, read the product label and fill in the information on each "product label" below. Then, answer the questions at the bottom of the page.

Supplement A

Type of supplement: _____

Brand name:_____

Recommended dosage: _____

Amount of key ingredient per dose: _____

Cost per dose: _____

Warnings: _____

_____

_____

Claims: _____

_____

_____

Supplement B

Type of supplement: _____

Brand name:_____

Recommended dosage: _____

Amount of key ingredient per dose: _____

Cost per dose: _____

Warnings: _____

_____

_____

Claims: _____

_____

_____

1. Describe any differences you noted between Supplement A and Supplement B. _____

_____

_____

_____

2. Why is it important to read the product label closely? _____

_____

_____

3. If you actually intended to purchase this type of supplement, would you choose Supplement A or Supplement B? Explain. _____

_____

_____

_____

4. Are either of the products you examined approved for use by the FDA? _____

5. How might the approval and regulation of the FDA make a supplement more safe?_____

_____

_____

_____

Backtrack
Through Chapter 23

Activity D

Chapter 23

Name _____

Date_____ Period _____

Provide complete answers to the following questions and statements about food and fitness trends.

Recall the Facts

1. How do food trends affect the food industry? _____

   _____

2. Name four current trends in the area of food and nutrition. _____

   _____

   _____

3. What types of ingredients make ethnic cuisines unique? _____

   _____

4. Name three types of businesses that provide home delivery of ready-to-eat meals. _____

   _____

5. How many adults in the United States are considered overweight? _____

6. From what is olestra made? _____

7. Which type of supplements account for the largest part of the growing market of supplements? _____

   _____

8. What side effects have been observed by people taking nonnutrient supplements? _____

   _____

9. What two main areas of scientific discovery will benefit food and nutrition in the future? _____

   _____

10. Name two synonyms for the word *bioengineering*. _____

11. How long does it take today to produce a plant with a desired trait through bioengineering? _____

    _____

12. In what three ways can bioengineering affect the future of nutrition and fitness? _____

    _____

13. What was the first bioengineered whole product? _____

Interpret Implications

14. Explain why reducing fat in the diet is so difficult. _____

    _____

    _____

(Continued)

Name_____

15. What statement in an ad for a nonnutrient supplement indicates the product has not been proven effective in doing what it claims? Why is the statement provided? _____

_____

_____

16. Explain how a vaccine creates an immunity. _____

_____

17. Explain how bioengineering is erasing the line between medicine and food. _____

_____

_____

18. Explain why irradiated foods are slow in coming to the market. _____

_____

Apply & Practice

19. Give three examples that reflect an inactive lifestyle. For each example, suggest how a person could make a change to become more active.

_____

_____

_____

_____

20. List five examples of products and services that have been produced by the fitness industry.

_____

_____

_____

_____

_____

_____

Nutrition and Health: A Global Concern

Meanings in Action

Activity A

Chapter 24

Name _____

Date _____ Period _____

Check your understanding of the meanings of key terms by trying to recognize the terms in action. In each set of terms and examples, match each term with the appropriate example. Write the letter of each answer in the space provided.

Group A: Countries

_____ 1. A country has a high economic level of living standards and industrial production.

_____ 2. A country has suffered droughts for the past three growing seasons and cannot grow enough food for its people.

_____ 3. A country has a rapidly growing birthrate and the farmland is no longer adequate to supply food for all the people.

A. developing

B. industrialized

C. overpopulated

D. underpopulated

Group B: Conditions

_____ 4. Twelve-year-old Sorina has lived on a low-protein diet since she was a baby.

_____ 5. A little boy died because he had nothing to eat or drink.

_____ 6. The people were very weak from a prolonged lack of food.

A. hunger

B. malnutrition

C. overnutrition

D. undernutrition

Group C: Access to Food

_____ 7. The people in a country lived on little more than potatoes for at least five years.

_____ 8. The country has a booming economy, and most of the people there have plenty of food.

_____ 9. The common people of the country have no food or water and are dying in large numbers.

A. famine

B. food insecurity

C. food security

D. starvation

Group D: Effects on People

_____ 10. Agnes weighs only 36 pounds, which is below the healthy range for her age.

_____ 11. Jeremy is only 4 feet 5 inches tall, well below the average height for a 15-year-old.

_____ 12. Philippe has lost over 30 pounds as his body tissues are being destroyed by disease.

A. stunted

B. subweight

C. underweight

D. wasted

(Continued)

Name_____

Group E: Statistics

_____13. The average value of goods and services produced went down each year during the last decade.

_____14. The number of infant and child deaths was decreasing.

_____15. The number of infants born each year was increasing.

A. birthrate

B. life expectancy

C. mortality rate

D. per capita GDP

Group F: Forms of Help

_____16. The church provides group meals for the elderly.

_____17. The volunteer group keeps food on the shelf for emergencies.

_____18. The soup kitchen receives mass-produced food items in bulk once a month.

A. commodity food

B. congregate meal

C. food pantry

D. food stamps

Group G: Beliefs and Actions

_____19. The general assembly passed a law on crop controls.

_____20. The country plans to expand its rice farming operations so it can export rice and sell it to other countries.

_____21. Lots of people believe that people go hungry because there is not enough food to go around.

A. cash crop

B. food policy

C. hunger legend

D. hunger myth

Group H: Solutions

_____22. The hunger coalition promotes the wise use of resources as the key to ending hunger.

_____23. The country has a good waterway and highway system, which is a real asset in economic development.

_____24. The celebrity spoke out on behalf of those who are hungry.

A. advocate

B. environmental sustainability

C. infrastructure

D. intrastructure

Group I: Programs

_____25. This program emphasizes the needs of children.

_____26. This program works to increase a nation's food supply.

_____27. This program focuses on fighting disease.

A. FAO

B. UNICEF

C. WHO

D. WIC

It All Adds up to Hunger

Activity B

Chapter 24

Name _____

Date_____ Period _____

The statistics listed below help depict the seriousness of world hunger. In the space beneath each one, write your response or interpretation of the statistic. What does it mean? What will be the results? Can these conditions affect you? If so, how? What would happen if these conditions described you, those around you, or the place you live? How would life be different?

1. The world's population is expected to jump from six billion to eight billion by 2025. _____
   _____
   _____

2. The average annual income in developing countries of South and East Asia and parts of Africa is less than $1,500 per person. _____
   _____
   _____

3. Many families in developing nations spend 80 to 90 percent of their income to buy food. _____
   _____
   _____

4. In the least-developed nations, 75 percent of the people die before they reach the age of 50._____
   _____
   _____

5. In developing countries, over 190 million children are underweight, 230 million are stunted, and 50 million are wasted. _____
   _____
   _____

6. About 30 to 70 million U.S. citizens lack nourishing food; safe, clean housing; and access to health care.
   _____
   _____

Which of these statistics did you find the most surprising? Explain. _____
_____
_____

Which of these statistics bothered you the most? Explain. _____
_____
_____

Name one thing you personally could do to help lower one of these statistics. _____
_____
_____

Hunger—Why Do I Care?

Activity C   Name _____

Chapter 24   Date_____ Period _____

Have you ever stopped to think about world hunger? Why might you care about the hunger problem? Make a list of these reasons. Check the appropriate block to indicate whether each reason is primarily humanitarian, political, or economic. Compare and contrast your list with those of classmates. Use the space at the bottom of the page to summarize the results.

Reasons	Humanitarian	Political	Economic

Summary of Findings:

_____

_____

_____

_____

_____

A Case in Point

Activity D

Chapter 24

Name _____

Date_____ Period _____

Use your media center or go online to research a country where hunger is a national problem. List existing conditions that are possible causes of hunger in that country. Place each condition in the appropriate category. Then in the space provided, write a letter to a government official in the country suggesting ways to address the problem.

Poverty

Overpopulation

Natural Disasters

Government Policies

Environmental Factors

Culture

Inadequate Education

(Continued)

Name_____

Dear _____,

_____
_____
_____
_____
_____
_____
_____
_____
_____
_____
_____
_____
_____
_____
_____
_____
_____
_____
_____
_____
_____
_____
_____
_____
_____
_____
_____

Signed, _____

Portrait of the Hungry

Activity E

Chapter 24

Name _____

Date_____ Period _____

Who are the people who are hungry? What traits describe them? Write descriptors around the sketch below to identify traits of hungry people. Use the left side of the sketch to list traits of hungry people in the United States. Use the right side to list traits of hungry people elsewhere around the globe. Compare and contrast descriptors used.

**Hungry People
in the United States**

**Hungry People
Around the World**

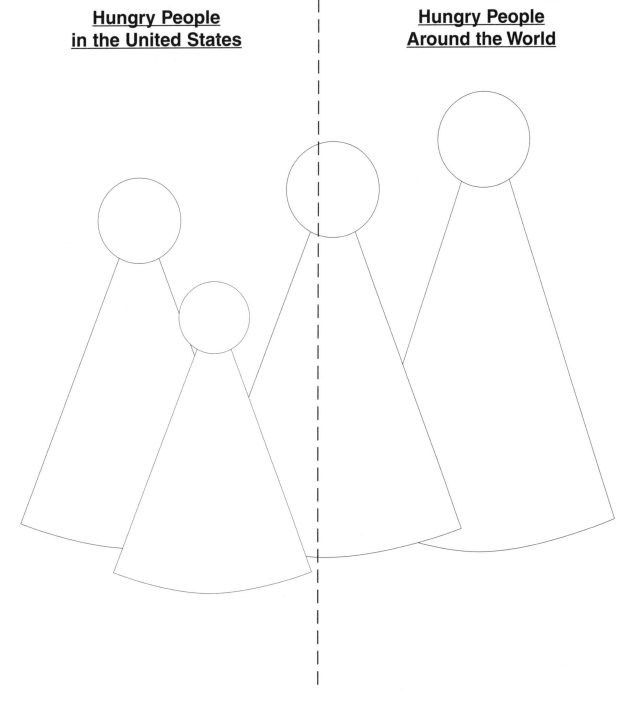

Stepwise Solutions to Hunger

Activity F   Name _____

Chapter 24   Date_____ Period _____

Hunger is a very complex problem. It must be attacked on each of five major fronts—economic, infrastructure, research and technology, population growth, and education. Each of the steps or strategies listed below is part of one of these fronts. Write each step or strategy inside the diagram of the front to which it belongs.

Steps/Strategies:

- Make food policies
- Improve schools
- Improve health
- Teach people to read
- Improve health education
- Teach job skills
- Improve waterways
- Teach gardening
- Improve highways

- Convert to market economies
- Improve nutrition
- Produce new food varieties
- Increase food yields
- Have a green revolution
- View hunger as an obstacle to growth

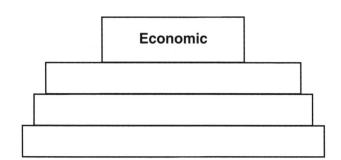

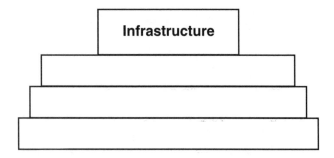

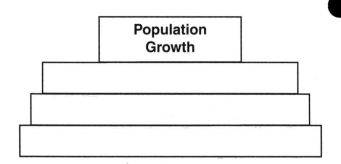

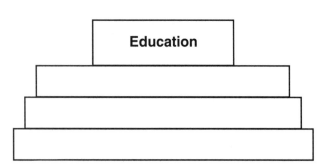

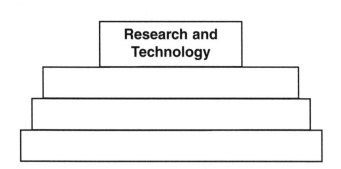

Backtrack
Through Chapter 24

Activity G

Chapter 24

Name _____

Date _____ Period _____

Provide complete answers to the following questions and statements about global concerns related to food and nutrition.

Recall the Facts

1. How many developing nations have been identified by the United Nations? _____

2. Where in the world are the greatest numbers of hungry people found?_____
_____

3. Compare the causes of famines in the past with those that occur today._____
_____
_____

4. What is the most common reason for global hunger today? _____

5. List five effects of malnutrition on young children. _____
_____

6. Name one of the nutrients the United Nations reports as deficient in the diets of developing countries and explain why a deficiency in this nutrient is a problem. _____
_____

7. Name six indicators used by the United Nations to profile the living conditions of people in different countries.
_____
_____
_____

8. Name three types of natural disasters that bring short-term hunger problems. _____
_____

9. What percentage of the population falls below the poverty line in the United States?_____

10. What worldwide effort turned many brown fields green? _____

11. When is World Food Day, and who sponsors it? _____
_____

Interpret Implications

12. Explain why some industrialized nations still face hunger problems. _____
_____

13. Explain why early weaning of children from breast milk causes such serious nutritional problems. _____
_____

(Continued)

Name_____

14. Briefly describe the poverty-malnutrition cycle._____

_____

_____

15. Explain why overpopulation affects the hunger problem. _____

_____

16. Explain why inadequate education is a factor in the hunger problem. _____

_____

17. Describe the extent to which the world's food resources are unevenly distributed. _____

_____

Apply & Practice

18. What is the current goal of the United Nations regarding world hunger? Do you think it will be reached? Why or why not? _____

_____

_____

_____

19. Write a paragraph describing why Americans should care about global hunger as well as hunger in the United States. _____

_____

_____

_____

_____

_____

_____

_____

_____

20. In the space below, write one of the hunger myths described in the text. Explain why you think people believe this myth and suggest one action that could be taken to dispel this myth. _____

_____

_____

_____

_____

_____

A Career for You in Nutrition and Fitness

Directions for Dietitians

Activity A

Chapter 25

Name _____

Date_____ Period _____

Read the following case situations about people who are dietitians or who plan to become dietitians. Answer the questions in the spaces provided. For all questions that ask about types of dietitians, select from among the following types: business, clinical, community, consultant, educator, management, and research.

Case #1—Hiram works as chief dietitian in a hospice facility. His job is to plan diets for individual patients and counsel family members about feeding practices for their loved ones.

    A. What type of dietitian is Hiram? _____

    B. Is Hiram a registered dietitian? _____ How do you know? _____

Case #2—Dara and Debbie were best friends in college. After graduation, Dara took a contract position with a nursing home where she advises the food service manager about diets for elderly patients. Debbie took a job as a dietetic consultant for a major supermarket chain. She advises supermarkets on what kinds of groceries to stock.

    A. What type of dietitian is Debbie? _____

    B. What type of dietitian is Dara? _____

Case #3—Sharon has always wanted to work in an educational setting. She has decided to develop her interest in nutrition by becoming a dietitian. She plans to go to college, get a bachelor's degree, and then look for a job immediately. Sharon does not want to pursue an advanced degree.

    A. Which two types of dietitians work in educational settings? _____

_____

_____

    B. Of these two types, which would be most compatible with Sharon's plans? Why? _____

_____

_____

Case #4—Carlos is a good public speaker. He is active in his community as a volunteer, and loves to work with people of all ages. Carlos is interested in nutrition and plans to major in dietetics at the local university.

    A. Would you recommend Carlos consider work as a research dietitian or a community dietitian? Why?

_____

_____

    B. How might he use his speaking ability as a dietitian? _____

_____

_____

Career Crossroads

Activity B

Chapter 25

Name _____

Date_____ Period _____

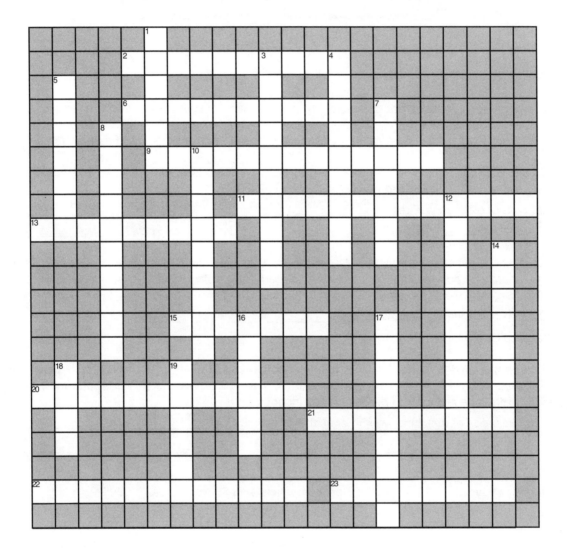

(Continued)

Name_____

Across

2. A _____ dietitian is certified and qualified to analyze a person's diet.
6. Taking steps to preserve your health now to prevent health problems later is _____ health care.
9. A competency that you need to get and keep a job is a(n) _____ skill.
11. A special standing within a profession achieved by meeting certain requirements is called _____.
13. People who graduate from a two-year program beyond high school earn a(n) _____ degree.
15. A work requirement set by a government agency is a _____.
20. A discussion between a job applicant and an employer is a(n) _____ .
21. A person who will speak highly of an individual's skills and abilities is a _____.
22. Someone who owns and operates a business is a(n) _____.
23. A person who completes about three to five years of school beyond the master's level earns a _____ degree.

Down

1. A bachelor's _____ is required for most careers in nutrition and fitness.
3. A job that requires few skills and pays minimal salary is _____.
4. A person who is trained to apply nutrition principles to diet planning is a(n) _____.
5. A person who completes a two-year program beyond the bachelor's level earns a(n) _____ degree.
7. A skill learned through practice is an _____.
8. Alerting a wide circle of people about an interest in a job is called _____.
10. An organized collection of materials showing what a person has accomplished is a(n) _____.
12. A dietetic _____ works under the direction of a registered dietitian.
14. A natural talent is a(n) _____.
16. Standards, guidelines, and codes that guide behavior are called _____.
17. The program of study that prepares a person to be a dietitian is called _____.
18. An aim you strive to reach is a(n) _____.
19. A fellow worker who has years of experience and can help with questions and challenges on the job is a(n) _____.

Nutrition and Fitness—A Story of Opportunity

Activity C

Chapter 25

Name _____

Date _____ Period _____

Complete this story by using context clues and your knowledge of career opportunities in nutrition and fitness. Write the missing words in the numbered blanks provided. Some choices may be used more than once, while others might not be used at all.

certified	director	exercise leader	science
corporate	enhancement	fitness	specialist
degree	entrepreneur	health	sports instructor
dietetic technicians	ergonomics	nutrition	untrained
dietitians	exercise	registered	

    The graduating class of Expectation High included 16 seniors who had taken Nutrition and Fitness as an elective course during their senior year. While taking the class, they had learned about the four main areas of career opportunity in the field of nutrition and fitness—(1) _____, (2) _____ _____, (3) _____ and (4) _____ specialists, and other food science professionals.

    Ten years later, Mr. Wellmann, the instructor, decided to do a follow-up survey to see how many of these 16 students had gone into careers related to his course of study. Wellmann learned 7 graduates were currently working in the nutrition and fitness field.

    Ginny Pollock was working as a(n) (5) _____ fitness specialist at an accounting firm called DuPre, Inc., where she directed a wellness program for the employees. She had worked at DuPre for two years.

    While she was in college, Mary Jumper worked part-time as a(n) (6) _____ _____ at the YMCA. There, she led two aerobic exercise classes per week. After she earned her degree in Exercise Science, she went back to the hometown YMCA and joined the staff as (7) _____ instructor, working one-on-one with individuals to provide counseling services for healthier lifestyles.

    Remembering that Jimmy Driskoll had always loved being in the lab during high school, Mr. Wellmann was not too surprised to learn he was now an exercise (8) _____ specialist in the Hastings Human Engineering Lab. His latest project was in the area of (9) _____, a study of human movement, in the business world.

    Yolanda Yetzin, who was on the swim team in high school, was now a (10) _____ _____ at the country club. She taught beginning and intermediate swimming lessons to both children and adults.

    Mr. Wellmann had received a letter several months earlier from Janet Lockley, CEHS. From the signature and return address, he knew Janet was working as a (11) _____ health education specialist at General Hospital. Since she was obviously certified, he knew she was also an RD or (12) _____ dietitian.

    Mr. Wellmann did not need to contact Anthony Burgaw. He had seen Anthony working at Downtown Park the last time he was there. When they talked, he remembered Anthony had worked in the park during high school as a(n) (13) _____ volunteer. Then he had gone to college, gotten his degree, and returned to the park to work full-time. Anthony had advanced to the top position of facility (14) _____.

    He also did not need to contact Adrienne Alston, who was now working at the high school as health (15) _____ instructor. She liked working with the high school students very much. Before working at the high school, Adrienne worked for three years as a(n) (16) _____ _____ at the Bounce-Back Rehabilitation Center. She helped patients regain their strength and coordination following illness or injury. She also helped them clarify (17) _____ misconceptions. Adrienne hopes to become a(n) (18) _____ in a few years, owning and operating her own business as a personal trainer.

Career Preparation Checklist

Activity D

Chapter 25

Name _____

Date_____ Period _____

Circle *Yes* or *No* to indicate whether you have done these steps in career planning. Use the comment space after each statement to write a note giving further details about your response. Then answer the questions at the end of the activity.

Yes   No   1. I have identified my interest in working with people, information, or material items.

Comment: _____

Yes   No   2. I have identified some careers that address my interest or overlapping interests.

Comment: _____

Yes   No   3. I am aware of my natural aptitudes—areas in which I often excel.

Comment: _____

Yes   No   4. I am working to develop abilities needed in my area of career interest.

Comment: _____

Yes   No   5. I have considered my career interests and options in light of my values.

Comment: _____

Yes   No   6. I have set long-term career goals and identified short-term goals that will help me reach them.

Comment: _____

Yes   No   7. I have taken (or am taking) courses that will prepare me for careers in my areas of interest.

Comment: _____

Yes   No   8. I have joined school or community organizations to develop my leadership and team-building skills.

Comment: _____

Yes   No   9. I have volunteered in a community service program that relates to my area of career interest.

Comment: _____

Yes   No   10. I am making a conscious effort to develop employability skills for career success.

Comment: _____

Yes   No   11. I have gained some work experience through part-time and/or summer jobs.

Comment: _____

Yes   No   12. I have talked with a counselor or someone who works in my area of career interest.

Comment: _____

Yes   No   13. I have begun to develop a portfolio that reflects my accomplishments.

Comment: _____

(Continued)

Name_____

Yes   No   14. I have begun to identify safe work environments where people work in my area of career interest.

Comment: _____

Yes   No   15. I have written a resume.

Comment: _____

Yes   No   16. I have located schools where I can study after high school in my area of interest.

Comment: _____

17. After answering the above questions, how well prepared do you think you are for your career search? Rate yourself using a scale from 1 to 10, with 1 being totally unprepared and 10 being very prepared. _____

Explain why you rated yourself as you did. _____

_____

_____

_____

18. Following the example of a mentor can help you maintain a job. Finding a mentor now can help you prepare to enter the world of work. What advice would you seek from a mentor as you prepare to begin your job search? _____

_____

_____

_____

19. Give an example of how you apply ethics in the school setting. Explain how this application is preparing you to use professional ethics in the workplace. _____

_____

_____

20. Do you have any interest in someday becoming an entrepreneur? Explain why or why not._____

_____

_____

_____

Practicing Interview Questions

Activity E

Chapter 25

Name _____

Date_____ Period _____

Take a few minutes to write your answers to these interview questions. Practicing your answers to frequently asked interview questions is a good way to prepare for an interview.

1. Where do you plan to be 10 years from now? _____
_____
_____

2. Why do you want to work in this career field? _____
_____
_____

3. What qualifications do you have for this position? _____
_____
_____

4. What do you know about our company, and why did you choose to apply here? ____
_____
_____

5. What is your greatest strength? _____
_____
_____

6. What is your greatest weakness? _____
_____
_____

7. What do you expect in the area of salary and benefits? _____
_____
_____

8. What was your best subject in school? _____
_____
_____

9. When will you be available to work? _____
_____
_____

10. Why should we hire you? _____
_____
_____

Backtrack
Through Chapter 25

Activity F

Chapter 25

Name _____

Date_____ Period _____

Recall the Facts

- -

Provide complete answers to the following questions and statements about careers in nutrition and fitness.

1. What is the minimum degree requirement for most nutrition and fitness professionals? _____

2. Select two of the career specialization areas for dietitians described in the text. Name one way these two specializations are alike and one way in which they are different. _____
   _____

3. What degree is generally required for work as a dietetic technician? _____

4. Select two of the career specialization areas for health and fitness specialists described in the text. Name one way these two specializations are alike and one way in which they are different. _____
   _____

5. What four types of requirements are generally set for certification and licensing in the field of nutrition and fitness? _____
   _____

6. Name three main influences that help shape a person's values. _____
   _____

7. Name three characteristics of effective goals. _____
   _____

8. Name eight high school courses that can prepare a person for a career in nutrition and fitness. _____
   _____
   _____

9. Name two organizations that foster leadership development for students in high school who are interested in nutrition and fitness. _____

10. List three points to keep in mind when selecting and listing references. _____
    _____

11. How should you dress for a job interview? _____
    _____

12. What are four traits that are often cited as keys to maintaining a job?_____
    _____

13. What are three key traits of successful entrepreneurs? _____
    _____

(Continued)

Interpret Implications

14. What could result if there were no certification or licensing regulations? _____
_____

15. Give two examples of aptitudes and two examples of abilities a person might have. _____
_____
_____
_____

16. Explain how sports and athletics can help a person prepare for a career in the fitness field. _____
_____
_____

17. Why is it important to behave professionally when leaving a job? _____
_____

Apply & Practice

18. List two examples of nutrition and fitness careers for people who like working with people, two for people who like working with information, and two for people who like working with material items.

People	Information	Material Items
_____	_____	_____
_____	_____	_____
_____	_____	_____

19. Identify two places in your community where people can volunteer in the fitness field. What types of tasks do volunteers perform in each place? _____
_____

20. Give an example of a specific workplace situation in which it would be important to display high standards of professional ethics. _____
_____
_____